An Atlas and Manual of

Cephalometric Radiography

Thomas Rakosi, M.D., D.D.S.
Professor of Orthodontics,
Chairman of the Orthodontic Department,
University of Freiburg.

Translated by **R. E. K. Meuss**

Wolfe Medical Publications Ltd

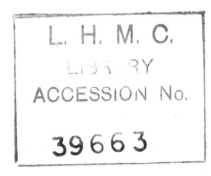
Originally published by Carl Hanser Verlag, Munich
as Atlas Und Anleitung Zur Praktischen
Fernröntgenanalyse/Thomas Rakosi.

© 1979 Carl Hanser Verlag

This book is one of the titles in the series of
Wolfe Medical Atlases, a series which brings
together probably the world's largest systematic
published collection of diagnostic colour photographs.
For a full list of Atlases in the series, plus
forthcoming titles and details of our surgical,
dental and veterinary Atlases, please write to
Wolfe Medical Publications Ltd, Wolfe House,
3 Conway Street, London W1P 6HE.

General Editor, Wolfe Medical Atlases:
G. Barry Carruthers, MD(Lond)

ISBN 0 7234 0767 3

This edition © 1982 Wolfe Medical Publications Ltd.

Printed in Great Britain by
Ebenezer Baylis & Son Ltd, Worcester.

Foreword

The use of cephalometric radiography in orthodontics serves to confirm diagnosis, and also makes it possible to include the morphology of the visceral cranium when considering possible treatment procedures. In the course of treatment, roentgenographic analysis can give valuable indications, by providing additional data when treatment is first initiated, a monitoring function as treatment progresses, and suggesting possible modifications. On conclusion of treatment it will often be the most important method for determining stability as well as the period of retention.

Cephalometric teleradiography will not, of course, replace any of the established methods of investigation. Radiographic diagnosis rather than analysis – i.e. making important therapeutic decisions wholly on the basis of radiographs – would indeed be poor diagnosis. To emphasize this point, the technique will always be referred to as 'cephalometric radiography' and not as 'diagnostic radiography'.

The method presented in this book is a practical one, i.e. designed for use in daily practice. A great number of analytical and investigatory procedures are specifically designed to assist scientific research. The present method also involves scientific researches but, if at all, these are mentioned only in passing.

A method designed for practical use must be based on meaningful measurements. All kinds of measurements may be made on a radiograph, but we are concerned only with parameters that provide the data needed for decision-making. Analysis is based on elements chosen with great care, based on the experience of many years. Its information value has been tested repeatedly, including the retrospective analysis of completed cases. For a period of two years, the work of our under-graduate, graduate and postgraduate students has been assessed and checked for accuracy by J. Jonas. Her conclusions have assisted us in the choice of landmarks. As exact definition of the different landmarks is of supreme importance, the chapter on "X-ray Anatomy" included in the present volume has been taken from her work.

In the planning of this book, didactic aspects were considered as well as the medical and scientific content. Its precursor entitled *Leitfaden für die Fernröntgenkurse* (manual for the courses in cephalometric radiography) was published in 1973. On the insistence of those who have attended our courses, the material from innumerable courses is now presented in concise form.

The introductory chapters discuss the general principles, X-ray anatomy, landmarks, lines and angles. This is followed by chapters on the significance of various skeletal, dental and soft tissue assessments. Two further chapters deal with the interpretation of results and of growth. Finally, practical examples are used to demonstrate treatment planning on the basis of radiological criteria. Countless examples could have been given to illustrate this chapter; the commonest form of malocclusion, the class II₁ anomaly, has been used to demonstrate the issues involved.

The conclusions drawn in that chapter show that the usefulness of cephalometric radiography is not limited to overall treatment planning. Every stage of treatment and innumerable technical details are in part planned on the basis of radiographic findings. Even what are considered simple procedures, such as determining the angle of traction for headgear, planning the construction bite or trimming the acrylic of an activator, cannot be effectively performed without radiological analysis.

The aim of the book is to integrate cephalometric radiography as far as possible with investigation and treatment planning in the field of orthodontics, to facilitate decision-making in daily practice, and enable the best form of treatment to be determined for each individual case.

Freiburg-im-Breisgau, Germany
August 1978   Th. Rakosi

Contents

Significance of Angular and Linear Measurements for Dento-Skeletal Analysis

Dento-Alveolar Analysis

Soft Tissue Analysis

Interpretation of Measurements

Cephalometric Radiography and Growth

Cephalometric Radiography in Treatment Planning

The Ranking Order of Cephalometric Radiography in Orthodontic Diagnosis

Cephalometry and Teleradiography

1 The Introduction of Cephalometry to Orthodontics

The assessment of craniofacial dimensions is not a new skill in orthodontics. The earliest method used was to assess facial proportions from an artistic point of view, with beauty and harmony as the guiding principles. Tastes change, however, and beauty was judged by different standards in antiquity than, for example, during the Renaissance. Dürer analysed the human face, determined the ideal proportions and divided the face into quadrants, and his work still has a bearing on orthodontics. Many centuries later, his method was applied to the analysis of cephalometric radiographs by de Coster and Moorees. Cephalometry (scientific measurement of the dimensions of the head) was the first method to prove of value in orthodontics. It was used to assess craniofacial growth and determine treatment responses. More accurate methods were based on oriented impressions of the face and dentures, an example being that of van Loon (*cubus craniophorus*). The method is demanding but very useful and was introduced under the name of 'gnathostatics' in 1922. A further method for the analysis of craniofacial dimensions that developed on the basis of cephalometry is cephalometric radiography.

The first X-ray pictures of the skull in the standard lateral view were taken by Pacini and Carrera (1922). In subsequent years, the following authors also produced this type of radiograph for the evaluation of craniofacial measurements: MacGowen (1923), Simpson (1923), Comte (1927), Riesner (1929), and others. None of them gave an accurate description of the methods used to take the pictures and for their evaluation, so that one can only speak of individual studies. It was not until 1931 that Hofrath and Broadbent simultaneously and independently developed standardised methods for the production of cephalometric radiographs, using special holders known as cephalostats, to permit assessment of growth and of treatment response.

Cephalometric radiography was introduced into orthodontics during the 1930s, but the method really only gained wider acceptance for practical application during the last twenty years. Over the years, a whole range of analyses has been developed by a number of authors. The aims of assessment tended to vary, ranging from studies on facial growth, the location of malformations, aetiological studies to the assessment of treatment response, as a complement to status analysis in orthodontics, etc. An analysis will only supply the answers to a particular set of questions, and these answers will depend on correct application of the method and interpretation of results. Over a hundred different analyses have been developed. They may be classified from a number of viewpoints, in systems devised by different authors.

For clinical application, the methods designed to assist diagnosis are of particular interest. The many different diagnostic analyses may be differentiated in a number of ways, according to the method of determination, the standards used, or the particular basis of analysis.

2 Classification of Analyses

2.1 Methodological Classification

The *basic units* of analysis are angles and distances in millimetres (lines). Measurements (in degrees or millimetres) may be treated as absolute or relative, or they may be related to each other to express proportional correlations.

2.1.1 Angular Analyses

The basic units are angle degrees.

2.1.1.1 *Dimensional analysis* considers the various angles in isolation, comparing them with average figures. Down's analysis is of this type (1948; Fig. 1a, b).

2.1.1.2 *Proportional analysis* is based on comparison of the various angles to establish significant relations between the separate parts of the facial skeleton. Koski's (1953) analysis belongs to this group, and this was developed further by Koski and Virolainon (1965). The results obtained with this analysis give the relations between the basic reference planes OP–N and OP–Pog in per cent (Fig. 2).

2.1.1.3 Analyses *to determine position*. Angular measurements may also be used to determine the position of parts of the facial skeleton. The SNA and SNB angles, for example, give the relations between the maxillary and mandibular bases and the cranial base.

Angular measurements on their own are not normally sufficient for cephalometry and linear measurements will be needed in addition.

Angular analyses have certain deficiencies:
The lines are drawn in relation to a primary reference plane, on the premise that this remains constant. If this plane shows deviations from the mean, the analysis is not reliable. Measurements are often related to particular norms or mean values. These norms are however subject to a number of factors, such as age, sex, hereditary and ethnic predisposition, etc. They are based on averages, and in the individual case it is the deviation from the mean that is characteristic.

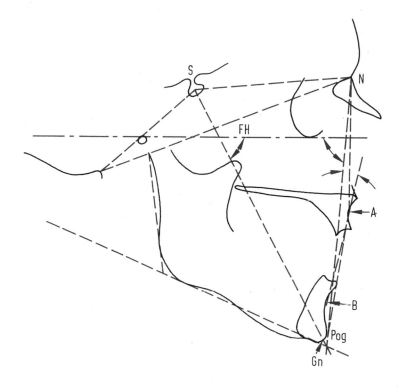

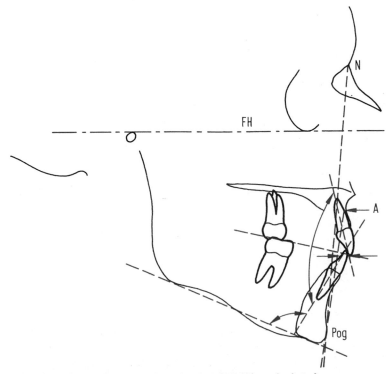

Fig. 1. Downs' dimensional angular analysis (1948), skeletal analysis; (b) Downs' dento-alveolar analysis.

2

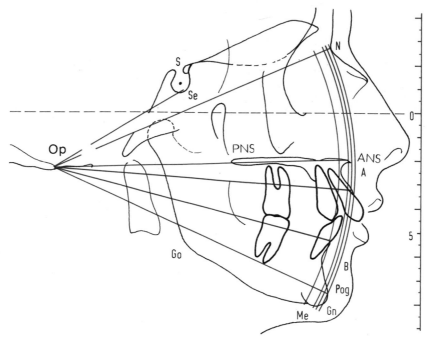

Fig. 2.   Proportional analysis of Koski and Virolainen (1956). This compares the different angles, to determine significant relationships between different parts of the facial skeleton.

2.1.2   Linear Analyses

For linear analysis, the facial skeleton is analysed by determining certain linear dimensions.

2.1.2.1   *Orthogonal analyses.* A reference plane is established, with the various reference points projected onto it perpendicularly, after which the distances between the projections are measured. Orthogonal analysis may be partial or total. *Total* orthogonal analysis may be geometrical or arithmetical. The de Coster method is a total orthogonal geometrical analysis (Fig. 3).

For the arithmetical method, the reference points are projected onto a horizontal and a vertical reference plane and the distances between the points on these planes determined (Fig. 4a, b).

Partial orthogonal analysis involves orthogonal assessment of only part of the facial skull. Willy (1947) for instance used the Frankfurt horizontal plane as the reference plane. He projected a number of reference points perpendicularly onto this, and measured the distances between the points thus obtained in the plane. The method differs from total orthogonal arithmetical analysis in that measurements are always made in one plane only.

2

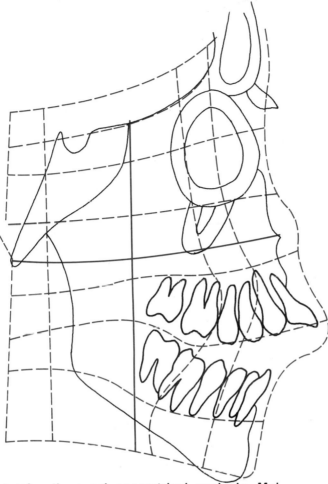

Fig. 3. de Coster's total orthogonal geometrical analysis. Malocclusion is demonstrated by deformation of the quadrants.

Orthogonal analyses are illustrative and suitable for teaching but not for diagnostic purposes. A further development of orthogonal methods are *archial analyses*, and these are a useful diagnostic aid.

The most widely known method is the Sassouni analysis (1958), with the reference points not projected perpendicularly, but by drawing arcs with the aid of compasses (Fig. 5).

2.1.2.2 *Dimensional, linear analyses* are based on evaluation of certain linear measurements, either direct or in projection.

The *direct* method gives certain linear measurements (e.g. the length of the mandibular base) as the distance between two reference points. The results are given in absolute terms, so that age also has to be taken into account for their interpretation.

Projected linear dimensional analysis determines the distances between certain reference points that have been projected onto a reference line.

2.1.2.3 *Proportional linear analyses* are based on relative rather than absolute values. The different measurements are compared to each other, without reference to norms.

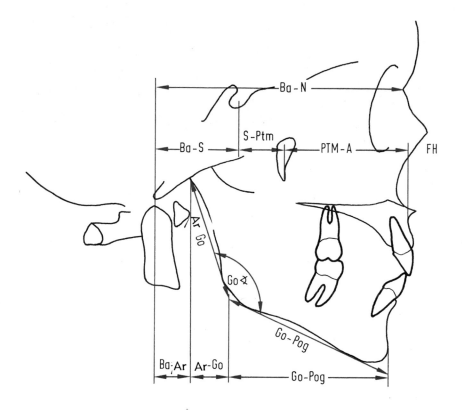

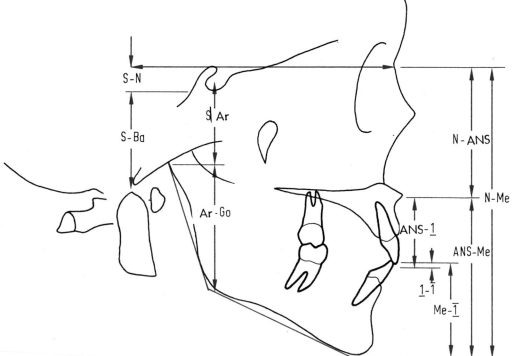

Fig. 4. Coben's total orthogonal arithmetical analysis assesses skeletal relationships parallel (a) and vertical (b) to the Frankfurt horizontal.

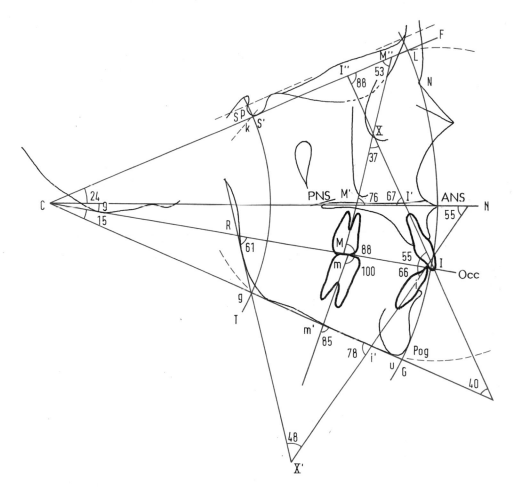

Fig. 5. Sassouni archial analysis. Landmarks are related not vertically, but by arcs drawn from a centre C.

2.2 Normative Classification

Analyses may also be classified according to the concepts on which normal values have been based.

2.2.1 Mononormative Analyses

Averages serve as the norms for these: they may be arithmetical or geometrical.

2.2.1.1 The *arithmetical norms* are average figures based on angular, linear or proportional measurements.

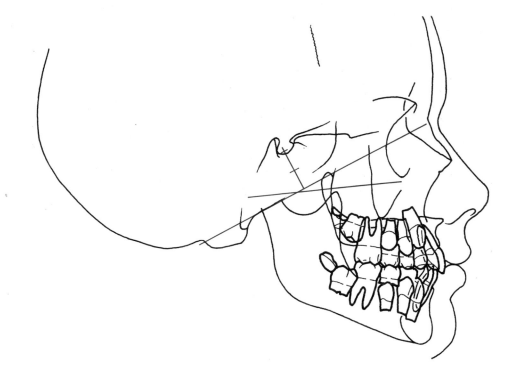

Fig. 6.   Average tracing of geometrical norms for children aged 10 (Bolton).

2.2.1.2   *Geometrical norms* are average tracings on a transparent sheet. Assessment consists in comparing these with the case under analysis. These methods merely provide rapid orientation (Fig. 6).

2.2.1.3   *The disadvantage of mononormative analyses* is that individual parameters are considered in isolation. Nor do they necessarily represent a 'normal' average, as deviations in the individual dimensions of the jaws and face may compensate each other so that occlusion is normal, just as 'normal' measurements may cumulatively tend to one end of the range of normal variation, the sum total being malocclusion. Mononormative analyses are suitable only for group studies, and not for diagnostic purposes.

2.2.2   Multinormative Analyses

For these, a whole series of norms are used, with age and sex taken into account (Tables 1 and 2).

2.2.3   Correlative Analyses

These are used to assess individual variations of facial structure to establish their mutual relationships. Correlative analyses are the most suitable for diagnostic purposes, and are used as such by most authors.

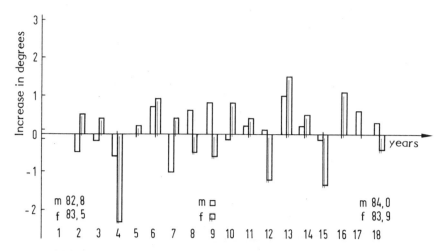

Table 1. Multinormative mean values for SNA angle. Age and sex analysis.

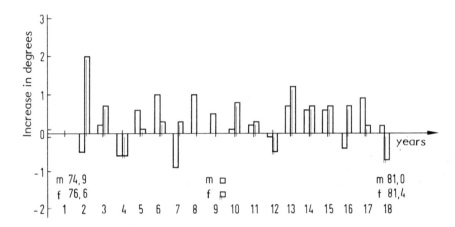

Table 2. Multinormative mean values for SNB angle. Age and sex analysis.

⊤ 2.3   Classification According to the Area of Analysis

The various analyses may involve limited areas or the whole of the facial skeleton.

2.3.1   Dentoskeletal Analyses

These analyze the teeth and skeletal structures. They may be made from norma lateralis, norma frontalis, or three-dimensionally. A more recent development is three-dimensional stereometric analysis, but this is not yet fully developed for clinical use.

2.3.2   Soft Tissue Analyses

These may involve the whole profile in norma lateralis, or certain structures only. We usually do a partial lateral soft tissue analysis, for example to analyse the lips in a cephalometric radiograph.

2.3.3 Functional Analyses

Cephalometric radiographs may also be used to assess functional relations such as the occlusion to interocclusal space relationship in norma lateralis and norma frontalis.

3 Producing the Cephalometric Radiograph

Cephalometric radiographs are produced at a considerable distance from tube target to Subject (2–4 metres), so that the visceral skull is correctly reproduced, without enlargement or distortion. The principal aim of the diagnostic analysis is to localise malocclusion within the content of the facial bone structures. Evaluation of the radiograph is based on standardised cephalometric landmarks.

The landmarks are used to determine lines and planes which then enable us to make linear and angular assessment of the radiograph.

4 Diagnostic Assessment of the Radiograph

Standards of general validity for diagnostic assessment do not exist. If an analysis does not reveal the nature of the anomaly under investigation this need not necessarily be due to inadequacies in the radiograph, but may arise because a method of assessment has been used that was not designed for that particular area of investigation. In clinical practice, evaluation of cephalometric radiographs is based on the principles given below.

4.1 Landmarks

Distinction is made between dentoskeletal and soft tissue points, and these may be unilateral (median) or bilateral. Depending on their origin, points may be anatomical, anthropological, or radiological (Fig. 7).

(1) In the median plane, unilateral points are located in the region of the cranial base, for instance in the midface and in the profile.

(2) Points located on either side and above the median plane result from superposition of two lateral points. The most important of these lie in the region of the mandible.

We prefer unilateral (situated in the median or sagittal plane) to bilateral points, as superposition of two points with bilateral location may involve loss of accuracy.

As far as possible, the points chosen are generally known points capable of being easily defined in a radiograph.

We have investigated the degree of personal error in the location of landmarks, and found (Jonas) that anatomical and also dental points are more reliable than constructed points.

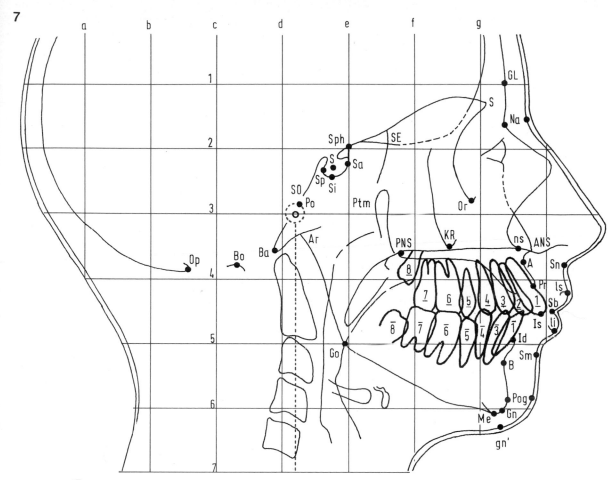

Fig. 7. Median and bilateral reference points used by Krogman and Sassouni.

4.2 Lines and Planes

Having located the points, we draw lines to mark the reference planes (Fig. 8). Linear measurements may be made by connecting two points, angular measurements between three points. Numerous lines are used in the different linear and angular analyses, with one particular line representing the reference plane on which the whole analysis is based. Two such planes are the Frankfurt horizontal plane and the sella-nasion. The Frankfurt horizontal plane, being based on bilateral points (orbitale and porion), is more subject to error. We therefore prefer the sella-nasion plane which is constructed with the aid of two median landmarks.

4.3 The Range of Analysis

Diagnostic analysis does not adhere to a rigid system. We do certain linear and angular measurements on a routine basis, but go beyond these in individual cases, depending on the nature of the anomaly, on the patient's age, and the method of treatment under consideration. Distinction is made between special and supplementary measurements.

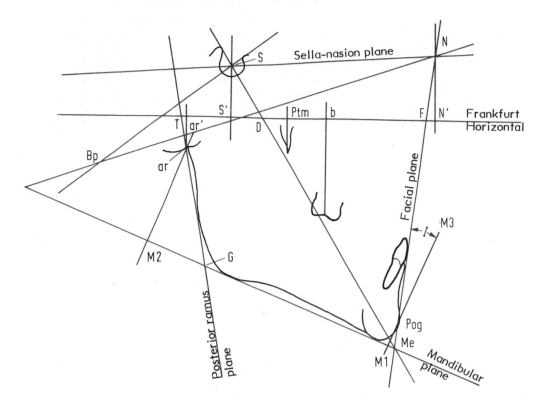

Fig. 8. **The most widely used reference lines.**

4.3.1 Control Measurements

These are made where the results of routine determinations leave room for doubt. We do, for example, make a routine analysis of the position of the upper incisors relative to the nasal spine and the SN plane. If the results are not unequivocal in either case as, for example, in cases of ante- or retroinclination, we make further measurements in order to get a clear picture. As far as possible, linear and angular measurements are used in combination.

4.3.2 Special Measurements

Special measurements are taken in individual cases where points of particular interest arise. An example would be the position of the sixth-year molars, which may be of considerable importance prior to and during headgear therapy (Fig. 9a, b and c).

4.3 Interpretation of Measurements

Individual measurements are considered not in isolation, but relative to each other. An unusually long mandibular base, for instance, does not in itself mean prognathism, but may be found with normal and even post-normal occlusion. What matters is the relationship between the mandible and the whole facial bone structure. Only correlative analysis will accurately localise a malocclusion within the context of the facial skeleton.

9a

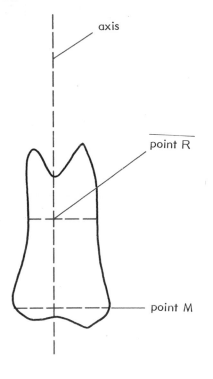

axis

point R

point M

9b

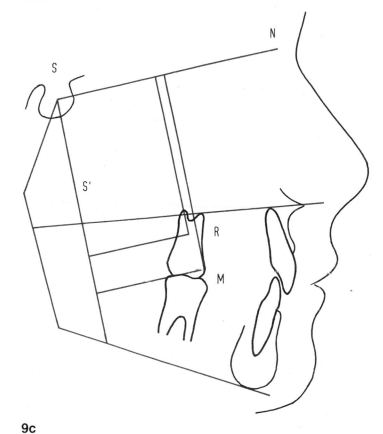

9c

Fig. 9. Special measurements to determine changes in 6th-year molar position. Reference points (a), diagrammatic representation of R and M vertical projection to give linear measurements (b), and diagrammatic representation of the angle between the axis of 6th-year molars and SN (c) to assess movement of the teeth.

X-ray Anatomy of the Visceral Cranium*

1 Norma lateralis

It is often difficult to establish a clear relationship between the size and shape of anatomical structures in the macerated skull on the one hand, and the contours seen in a lateral teleradiograph on the other. The differences are due to the technique used – i.e. the laws of central projection – and to representing a three-dimensional structure in two dimensions. Interpretation is made more difficult by differences in density, or contrast of the projected structures.

Exact location of the anatomical landmarks used in cephalometric radiology will require adequate knowledge of the X-ray appearance of the cranial bones and their relationship to adjacent structures.

Numerous features are discernible, such as lines – the projection of bony structures, shadows – representing soft tissues, and large radiolucent areas – indicating pneumatisation.

Below, a series of radiographs and outline drawings are given to facilitate general orientation. This will be followed by a more detailed discussion of areas of particular relevance to cephalometric radiography. The figures given in brackets correspond to those in Figs. 10 to 16.

2 Bony Outlines in the Radiograph

In Fig. 10a, b, the bony outlines consistently seen in X-ray pictures have been traced. Their radiodensity may of course vary.

Moving from above to below in the anterior part, there are the following: The anterior wall of the frontal sinus (1), the nasal bone (2), the frontal process of the maxilla (3), the anterior wall of the maxillary sinus (4), the floor of the nose, the alveolar process of the maxilla (7), and the anterior aspect of the mandible.

In the middle part of the picture, the following structures may be discerned: the roof of the orbit (8), with the opaque line continuing into the planum sphenoidale (12), the cribriform plate of the ethmoid bone (10), and the upper and lower limits of the maxillary sinus.

Posteriorly the X-ray shows: The hypophyseal fossa in profile (13), its dorsal limit continuing into the clivus (14). Below the most caudal part of the clivus – the basion (14a) – the shadow of the dens axis (15) may be seen, and mesial to it a smaller, more or less triangular outline representing the anterior arch of the atlas (16).

Ventrally to these structures, the condylar process of the mandible (17) is visible; it continues forwards into the mandibular incisure and finally the coronoid process (18).

Being very similar to the macerated skull, the body and ramus of the mandible is easily distinguished.

Some of the soft tissue outlines commonly seen in lateral views have also been traced. The soft palate is outlined, with the uvula (19), and the shadow of the posterior wall of the nasopharynx (20).

*From J. Jonas, *Mathematisch-statische Erhebung über die Grössenordnung des individuellen Fehlers in der Röntgenkephalometrie.* Freiburg, 1975.

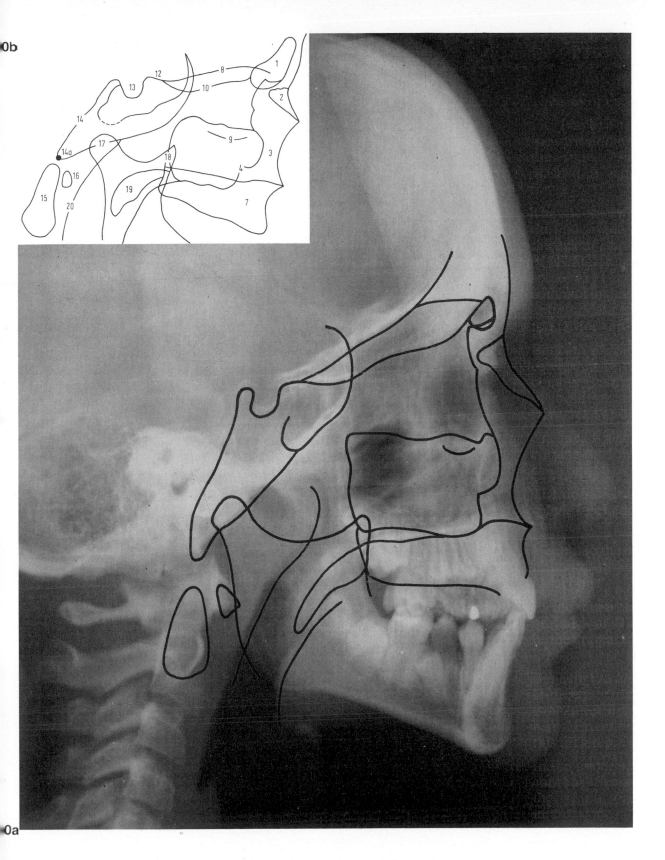

Fig. 10.   Bony contours in the radiograph. (a) In the radiograph,
(b) diagrammatic.

3 Paranasal Sinuses

Fig. 11a, b shows the air-filled spaces in the skull. These are subject to individual variation and their X-ray appearance also depends on the degree of pneumatisation: Frontal sinus (21), sphenoidal sinus (22), ethmoidal air cells (23), maxillary sinus (24) and nasopharyngeal space (25).

The lowest point of the frontal sinus is at the height of the nasion, the anterior upper end of the frontonasal suture. Its supraorbital recess (28 in 12a, b) may have pushed apart the lamina interna and orbitalis of the inner table of the frontal bone.

The ethmoidal air cells (23) lie between the frontal cells and the body of the sphenoid bone. Their lower limit is the roof of the maxillary sinus, the cranial limit the cribriform plate of the ethmoid bone.

The margins of the ethmoid bone are not easily defined because of its great variability. The anterior air cells may be masked by the frontal process of the maxilla. The middle cells with the ethmoidal bulla lie behind the zygomatic bone, and the posterior wall of the sinus is masked by the shadow of the greater wing of the sphenoid.

The sphenoidal sinus (22) lies immediately below the sella turcica and usually has a number of components. Ventrally and caudally it extends beyond the floor of the middle cranial fossa. Anteriorly, the planum sphenoidale forms its roof.

The nasopharyngeal space (25) lies between the shadow of the soft palate and the upper part of the posterior wall of the pharynx. It connects with the oral cavity. At the top, the space is limited by a line that is a radiological artefact, a projection of the posterior edge of the vomer. This is however masked by the shadow of the pterygoid process which also covers the posterior part of the superior meatus of the nose, so that the latter is only rarely identifiable.

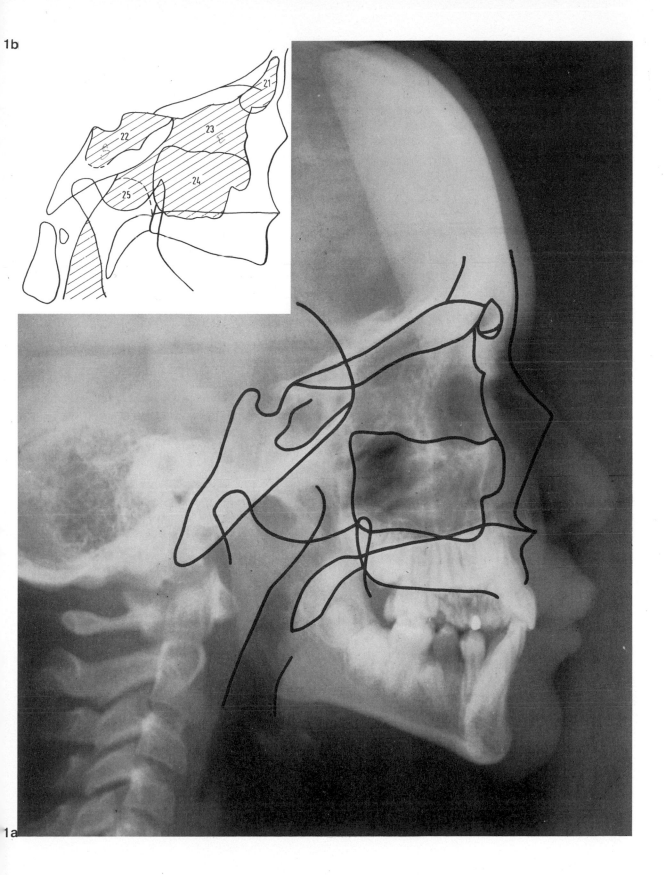

1b

1a

Fig. 11.   Paranasal sinuses. (a) In the radiograph, (b) diagrammatic.

The X-ray appearance of structures difficult to identify because of the numerous lines seen in the radiograph is discussed below.

4 The Roof of the Orbit

In the upper part of Fig. 12a, b, the floor of the anterior cranial fossa is traced. This is formed bilaterally by the roof of the orbit (8) and in the median by the cribriform plate of the ethmoid (10) and the planum sphenoidale (12).

The roof of the orbit (8) produces a dense outline, usually a double structure, due to its being bilateral. It merges dorsally into the planum sphenoidale (12), almost a straight line, and divides into two less marked structures ventrally. The upper one goes in a cranioventral direction, forming a dorsally concave line; the other one tends in a more downward direction, running into the shadow of the cribriform plate (10).

Some pointed elevations are distinguishable in the region of the orbital roof – these represent the cerebral ridges (26).

The external surface of the frontal bone terminates with an anteriorly convex curve in the frontonasal suture (30). Krogman and Sassouni (1957) state that because the caudally adjoining nasal bone (2) differs in radiodensity, it is not always easy to determine the uppermost point of the frontonasal suture. There is a risk of putting this point too far in the dorsal region. Overlap with the eyelids in this area may produce another fine structure that could be confused with the suture.

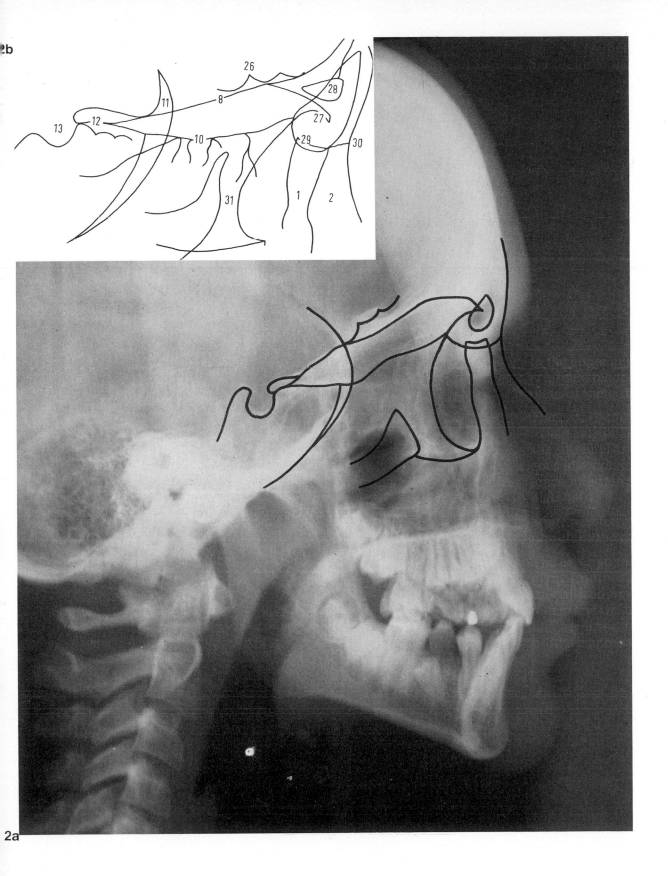

Fig. 12. Roof of orbit. (a) In the radiograph, (b) diagrammatic.

5 The Sphenoid Bone

Fig. 13a, b: The outline of the sella turcica, convex to the vertex, stands out clearly from its surroundings on every radiograph. It terminates in the tuberculum sellae (34) anteriorly and in the dorsum sella (35) posteriorly. As it is elliptical, a double line is often seen in this area. According to van der Linden (1971), the most radio-opaque lines represent the median or sagittal plane. The most caudal line is the floor of the sella, and the most dorsal shadow the median of the dorsum sellae (35).

The image of the tuberculum sellae (34) is frequently masked by the anterior clinoid processes so that the anterior limit to the entrance of the sella is not always clearly discernible. It does however stand out from the surrounding structures because it shows continuous transition into the line representing the floor of the sella, with its shadow denser than those of the anterior clinoid processes (van der Linden, 1971).

The lesser wing (33) shows as a line beneath the tuberculum sellae (34) which may show downward crenations indicating the optic canal. The upper part originates in the anterior clinoid processes (36) and continues in a ventral direction parallel to the planum sphenoidale (12), finally becoming tangential to the shadow of the greater wing. As already mentioned, the outlines of the lesser wing of the sphenoid are less radio-opaque than those of the adjacent planum sphenoidale and of the greater wing.

Dorsal to the cribriform plate of the ethmoid bone, the greater wing of the sphenoid appears in relief, its facies cerebralis forming a dense broad line that continues in a ventrally concave arc across the floor of the anterior cranial fossa, moving dorsocaudally. It produces a double contour in this area, the facies cerebralis interna (38) and the facies orbitalis (39). The facies temporalis (40) may sometimes be visible in the region of the anterior sphenoidal sinus (22).

The contour of the dorsum sellae (35), the posterior limit of the fossa hypophysialis, continues dorsocaudally into the shadow of the clivus (14) which consists of the body of the sphenoid and the basilar part of the occipital bone. The shadow extends from its more caudal point, the basion, cranioventrally to the anterior lower part of the sphenoid. Across the broad shape of the clivus, the faintly sketched line of the sphenooccipital synchondrosis (42) runs from dorsocranial to ventrocaudal.

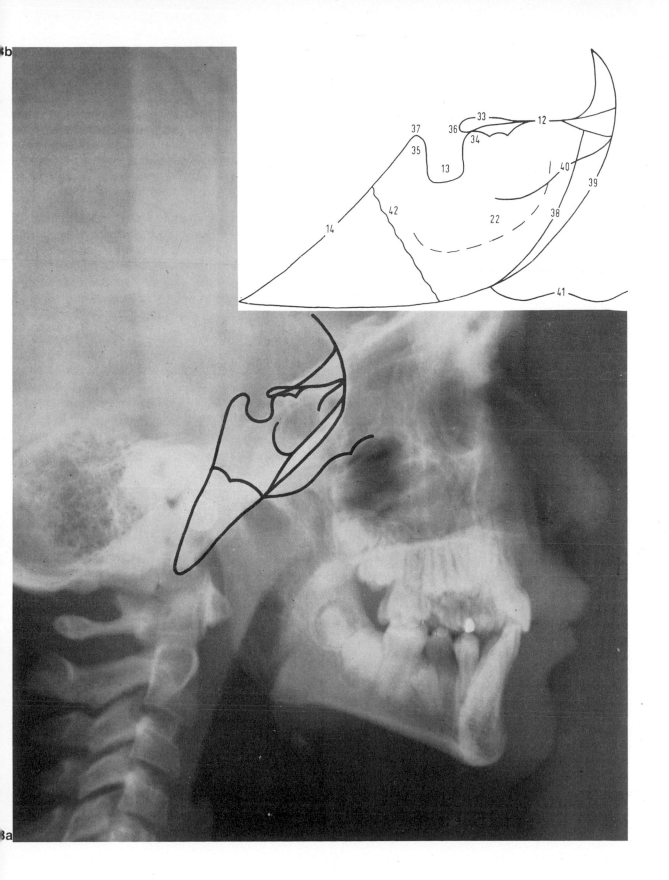

Fig. 13.   Sphenoid bone. (a) In the radiograph, (b) diagrammatic.

6   The Maxillary Sinus

The size of the maxillary sinus depends on the degree of pneumatisation.

Fig. 14a, b: The anterior wall of the sinus (4) is usually clearly distinguishable from the surrounding structures. It extends upwards and back to form the upper limit of the maxillary sinus. This line is rather delicate and tends to be irregular. It is partly masked by the ethmoidal air cells (23) and therefore not completely visible at times.

The shadow of the anterior wall of the sinus continues downwards and back into the floor of the sinus. The caudal part of a normally developed sinus extends below the palatine process of the maxilla (6) which forms a long, dense line running more or less horizontally across the picture, terminating ventrally in the anterior nasal spine (43). According to Hunter (1968), superposition of anatomical contours is common in this area due to the alae cartilagenes nasales, and it is possible to put the anterior nasal spine, the most caudal and anterior point of the piriform aperture, too far forward.

Beneath the latter, the external anterior limit of the maxilla forms an anteriorly convex curve running down to the alveolar border of the central incisors. This contour is not always very radio-opaque, and with poor contrast one runs the risk of localising the deepest retraction of the curve too far in the distal direction (Krogman and Sassouni, 1957).

The area is also masked by the soft tissues of the cheek. This produces an outward curving shadow in the region of the anterior limit of the maxillary base, and may cause mistakes in locating point A.

The dorsal limit of the palatine process (6) is represented by the posterior nasal spine. In children, this may frequently be masked by the images of unerupted molars.

Ventral to the maxillary sinus lies the frontal process of the maxilla (3). Depending on contrast, this may be more or less clearly distinguishable from the contour of the nasal bone.

In the upper anterior section of the maxillary sinus appears the contour of the orbital floor (9); dorsal to this shadow are two approximately parallel lines running in the cranial direction – the anterior and posterior limits of the zygomatic bone (31).

Beneath the orbital floor (9) an opaque, roughly triangular structure may be seen. Different opinions are given in the literature as to which specific bone this belongs. Bouchet et al. (1955) considers these structures to form part of the zygomatic bone, whilst Etter (1970) used radiological studies on isolated bones to demonstrate that this area represents mainly the zygomatic process of the maxilla (44).

In the upper part of the posterior maxillary sinus, the outline of the middle nasal concha (45) may be noted. This appears as a shadow clearly rounded at the back. If the inferior nasal concha (46) is hypertrophied, it may be located beneath the middle concha.

The coronoid process of the mandible (18) lies within the lower part of the sinus outline, but its contours are rather indistinct.

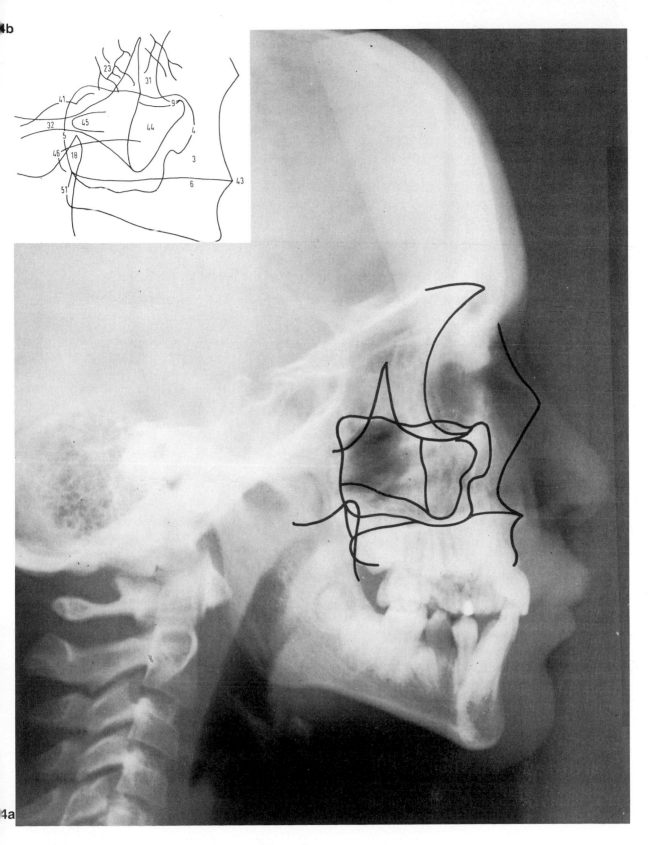

**Fig. 14. Maxillary sinus. (a) In the radiograph, (b) diagrammatic.
(See text, page 28.)**

29

7 The Pterygopalatine Fossa

The contour of the pterygopalatine fossa is a roughly triangular shape ending in a sharp point caudally.

Fig. 15a, b: Its upper limit is formed by the sphenomaxillary surface of the greater wing (41). The medial pterygoid plate (48) is its posterior wall whilst ventrally it is limited by the posterior wall of the maxillary sinus (5), a clearly visible line that continues caudally into the maxillary tuberosity (51). The contours of the zygomatic arch (32) and caudal to it the coronoid process of the mandible (18) cut across the upper part of the pterygopalatine fossa. The shadow of the foramen rotundum (47) appears in the cranial part.

The caudal extension of the anterior part of the fossa intersects with the contour of the floor of the nose and the soft palate. Compared to the macerated skull the fissure is situated in the transverse plane, at the same height as the posterior nasal spine.

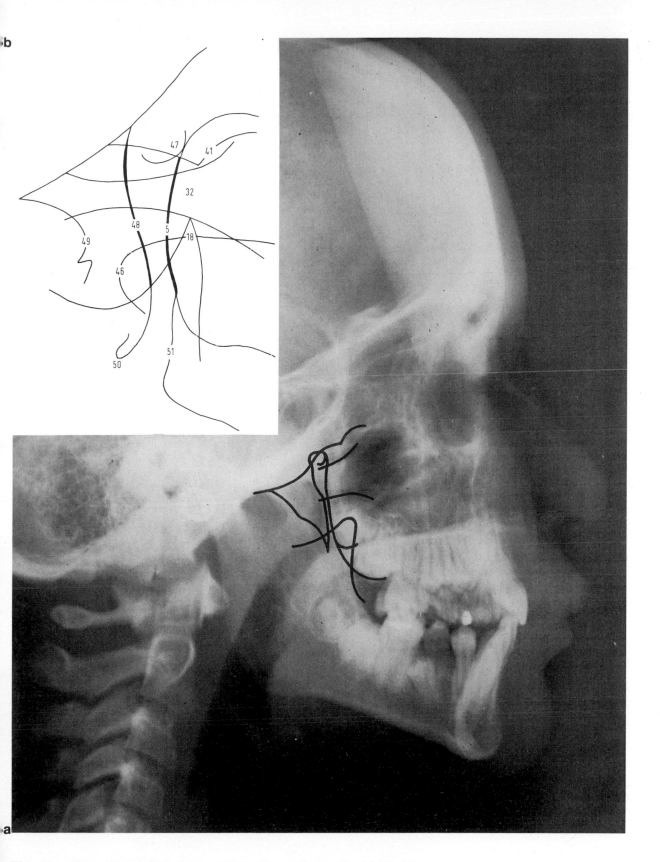

Fig. 15. Pterygopalatine fossa. (a) In the radiograph, (b) diagrammatically.

8 The Middle Cranial Base

In the middle region of the base of the skull, interpretation of contours is made difficult by the multiplicity of superposed structures. The area is also subject to considerable individual and age-related variation.

Fig. 16a, b: In the upper anterior part of the diagram lies the contour of the sphenoid bone, with the sella turcica (13) continuing downwards and back to the clivus (14).

Dorsal to the clivus is the upper inner margin of the petrous part of the temporal bone (52).

The region below this has a broken up, cloudy appearance due to the air-filled mastoid cells.

In the lower part of the diagram, the following contours are shown, moving from the anterior to the posterior parts: The zygomatic arch (32), the articular tubercle (53), and the condylar process of the mandible (17) which borders onto the image of the mandibular fossa.

Basion, the most caudal point of the clivus (14), is the most anterior edge of the foramen magnum, the lateral border of which is the occipital condyles (54). Their image appears close to the dens of the axis (15), forming a line that becomes more horizontal at its lower edge and continues dorsally into the condylar fossa (55).

Across the shadow of the occipital condyles lies the contour of the mastoid process (56).

From about the age of 14 onwards, the mastoid process extends caudally beyond the condyles. For differential diagnosis, its arc is more strongly convex to the cranium than the condyles, and it may also be located by the mastoid air cells.

Dorsal to the lower part of the clivus (14) lies the opening of the external acoustic meatus (57), an approximately circular shape, and dorsocranial to it the smaller contour of the opening to the internal acoustic meatus.

If ear olives are used with the cephalostat, the external acoustic meatus presents as a completely radio-opaque structure.

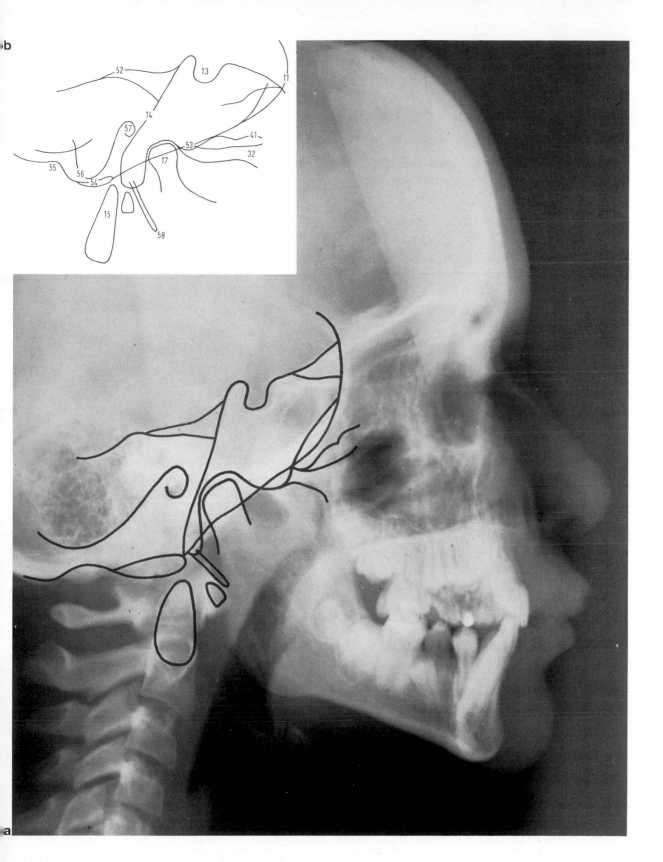

Fig. 16. Middle cranial base. (a) In the radiograph, (b) diagrammatically (see text, page 32).

Landmarks

1 Reference Points

The effective evaluation of radiographs depends on accurate definition and localisation of landmarks, which provide the basis for all further work.

Distinction is made between *anatomical* and *anthropological* points which are located on or within the skeletal structures.

Radiological or *constructed* points are secondary landmarks marking the intersections of X-ray shadows or lines.

1.1 Properties of Reference Points

1.1.1 Ease of Location

According to Moyers (1973), this depends on the following factors:

1.1.1.1 *Quality of the radiograph*. The quality of the picture is often marred by magnification or distortion.

Magnification is due to divergence of the X-rays. The smaller the focus-film distance and the greater the object-image distance, the greater is the magnification.

Distortion arises from two-dimensional representation of a three-dimensional object. All elements not in the image plane are subject to distortion. Accurate centring and positioning of the head will largely eliminate it. The median or sagittal plane of the head must be parallel and the central ray perpendicular to the film.

1.1.1.2 *Overlapping anatomical contours*. Facial structures overlap a great deal (see X-ray Anatomy, page 23), so that the location of certain landmarks may present problems. Such radiological peculiarities need to be taken into account in the selection of landmarks.

1.1.1.3 *Observer experience*. Observer experience and practice play a major role in the interpretation of radiographs, with knowledge of anatomy and X-ray anatomy as a key factor.

1.1.2 Constancy of Contours

The structures of the skull show dependence on a number of factors such as age, sex, growth, race, etc. The constancy of contours is therefore not entirely reliable in contradistinction to points located close to the base of the skull, where variation due to growth is minimal (e.g. nasion and sella).

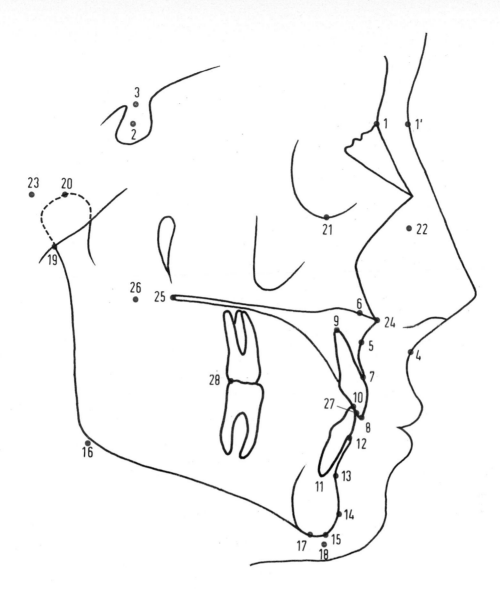

Fig. 17. Reference points used on a routine basis.

1.2 Definition of Reference Points

The points we use on a routine basis are shown in Fig. 17. Our definition of them is as follows:

No.	Code	Definition
1	N	*Nasion*. The most anterior point of the nasofrontal suture in the median plane. The skin nasion (N¹) is located at the point of maximum convexity between nose and forehead (Fig. 18).
2	S	*Sella*. We use the midpoint of the sella (S) in our analysis, and also the midpoint of the entrance to the sella (Se), after A.M. Schwarz. The sella point (S) is defined as the midpoint of the hypophysial fossa. It is a constructed (radiological) point in the median plane.

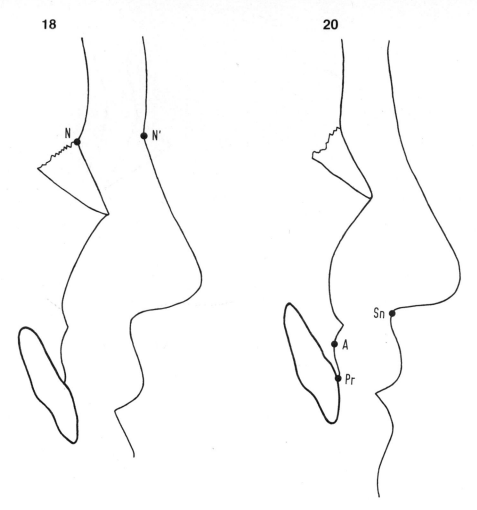

Fig. 18.   Nasion and soft tissue nasion.   **Fig. 20.   Subnasale, point A and prosthion.**

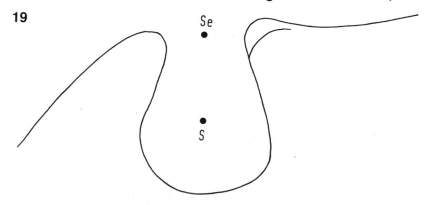

Fig. 19.   Localisation of S and Se.

3   Se   *Midpoint of the entrance to the sella*, according to A.M. Schwarz at
the same level as the jugum sphenoidale, independent of the
depth of the sella. This point represents the midpoint of the line
connecting the posterior clinoid process and the anterior opening
of the sella turcica (Fig. 19).

4   Sn   *Subnasale*. A skin point; the point at which the nasal septum
merges mesially with the integument of the upper lip (Fig. 20).

5	A	*Point A, subspinale*. The deepest midline point in the curved bony outline from the base to the alveolar process of the maxilla, i.e. at the deepest point between the anterior nasal spine and prosthion. In anthropology, it is known as subspinale (Fig. 20).
6	APMax	The *anterior* landmark for *determining the length of the maxilla*. It is constructed by dropping a perpendicular from point A to the palatal plane.
7	Pr	*Prosthion*. Alveolar rim of the maxilla; the lowest, most anterior point on the alveolar portion of the premaxilla, in the median plane, between the upper central incisors (Fig. 20).
8	Is (or Is$\underline{1}$)	*Incisor superius*. Tip of the crown of the most anterior maxillary central incisor.
9	Ap$\underline{1}$	*Apicale $\underline{1}$*. Root apex of the most anterior maxillary central incisor.
10	Ii (or Is$\overline{1}$)	*Incisor inferius*. Tip of the crown of the most anterior mandibular central incisor.
11	Ap$\overline{1}$	*Apicale $\overline{1}$*. Root apex of the most anterior mandibular central incisor.
12	Id	*Infradentale*. Alveolar rim of the mandible; the highest, most anterior point on the alveolar process, in the median plane, between the mandibular central incisors (Fig. 21).
13	B	*Point B, supramentale*. Most anterior part of the mandibular base. It is the most posterior point in the outer contour of the mandibular alveolar process, in the median plane. In anthropology, it is known as supramentale, between infradentale and pogonion (Fig. 21).
14	Pog	*Pogonion*. Most anterior point of the bony chin, in the median plane (Fig. 21).

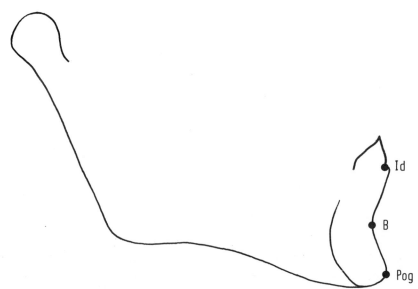

Fig. 21.   Infradentale, point B and pogonion.

15 Gn *Gnathion.* This point is defined in a number of ways. According to Martin and Saller (1956), it is located in the median plane of the mandible, where the anterior curve in the outline of the chin merges into the body of the mandible. Many authors have located gnathion between the most anterior and the most inferior point of the chin. Graig defines it with the aid of the facial and the mandibular plane; according to Graig, gnathion is the point of intersection of these two planes. Muzi and May give it as the lowest point of the chin (A.M. Schwarz uses the same definition) and therefore synonymous with Menton (Fig. 22).

Our own definition of gnathion is as the most anterior and inferior point of the bony chin. It is constructed by intersecting a line drawn perpendicularly to the line connecting Me and Pog with the bony outline.

16 Go *Gonion.* A constructed point, the intersection of the lines tangent to the posterior margin of the ascending ramus and the manibular base (Fig. 22).

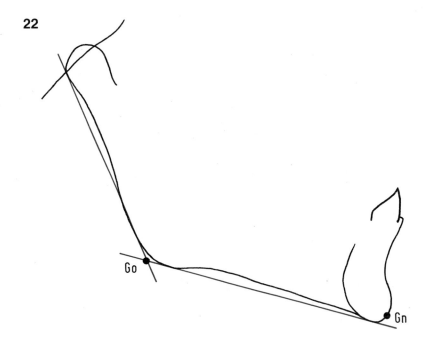

Fig. 22.   Gonion and gnathion.

17 Me *Menton.* According to Krogman and Sassouni, Menton is the most caudal point in the outline of the symphysis; it is regarded as the lowest point of the mandible (Fig. 23) and corresponds to the anthropological gnathion.

18 APMan The *anterior* landmark for *determining the length of the mandible.* It is defined as the perpendicular dropped from Pog to the mandibular plane.

19	ar	*Articulare*. This point was introduced by Bjork (1947). It provides radiological orientation, being the point of intersection of the posterior margin of the ascending ramus and the outer margin of the cranial base (Fig. 24).
20	Cd	*Condylion*. Most superior point on the head of the condyle (Fig. 24).
21	Or	*Orbitale*. Lowermost point of the orbit in the radiograph (Fig. 25).
22	Pn/2	*A constructed point*. It is obtained by bisecting the Pn vertical, between its intersection with the palatal plane and point N'.
23	Int.FH/ R.asc.	*Intersection* of the ideal Frankfurt horizontal and the posterior margin of the ascending ramus.

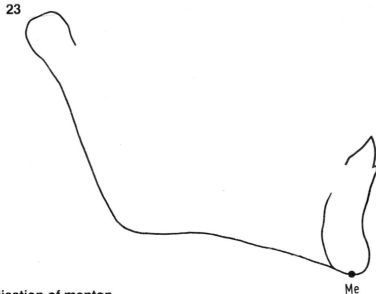

Fig. 23. Localisation of menton.

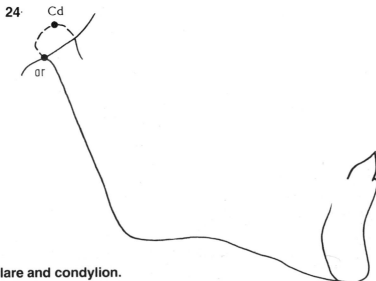

Fig. 24. Articulare and condylion.

24 ANS *Anterior nasal spine*. Point ANS is the tip of the bony anterior nasal spine, in the median plane (Fig. 25).
It corresponds to the anthropological acanthion.

25 PNS *Posterior nasal spine*. This is a constructed radiological point, the intersection of a continuation of the anterior wall of the pterygo-palatine fossa and the floor of the nose. It marks the dorsal limit of the maxilla (Fig. 25).

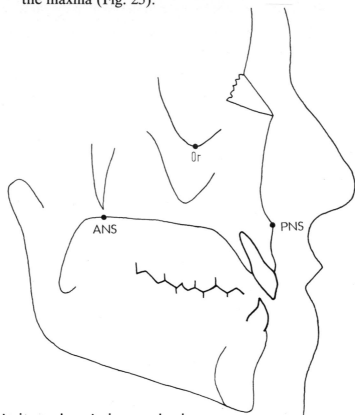

Fig. 25. Orbitale, anterior and posterior nasal spine.

26 S′ *Landmark* for assessing the length of the maxillary base, in the posterior section. It is defined as a perpendicular dropped from point S to a line extending the palatal plane.

27 APOcc *Anterior point for the occlusal plane*. A constructed point, the midpoint in the incisor overbite in occlusion.

28 PPOcc *Posterior point for the occlusal plane*. The most distal point of contact between the most posterior molars in occlusion.

We also use the following landmarks (see Fig. 7 and 8).

29 Ba *Basion*. Lowest point on the anterior margin of the foramen magnum in the median plane.

30 Ptm *Pterygomaxillary fissure*. The contour of the fissure projected onto the palatal plane. The anterior wall represents the maxillary tuberosity outline, the posterior wall the anterior curve of the pterygoid process.

This point corresponds to PNS.

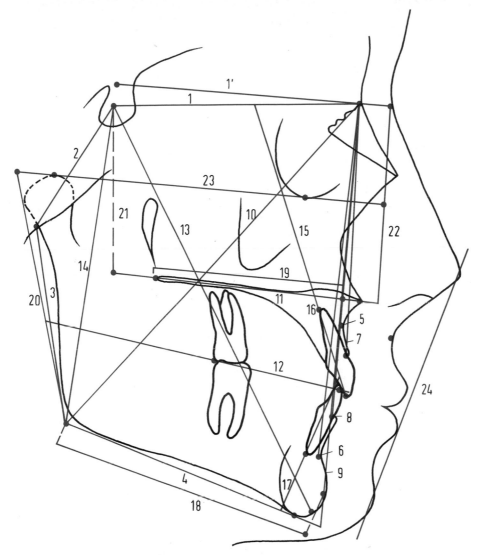

6

Fig. 26. Reference lines used in our analysis.

2 Reference Lines

The points described above are used to construct a considerable number of lines. Below is a description of the lines we most frequently use (Fig. 26).

No.	Line	Definition
1	S-N (Se-N)	Sella-nasion. Anteroposterior extent of anterior cranial base
2	S-Ar	Lateral extent of cranial base
3	ar-Go	Length of ramus (1st measurement)
4	Me-Go	Extent of mandibular base (1st measurement)
5	N-A	Nasion – point A

6	N-B	Nasion – point B
7	N-Pr	Nasion – prosthion
8	N-Id	Nasion – infradentale
9	N-Pog	Nasion – pogonion
10	N-Go	Nasion – gonion line, for analysis of the gonial angle
11	Pal	Palatal plane (ANS-PNS)
12	Occ	Occlusal plane (APOcc-PPOcc)
13	S-Gn	Y-axis
14	S-Go	Posterior facial height
15	1-SN	Long axis of upper incisor to SN
16	1-Pal	Long axis of upper incisor to Pal
17	1-MP	Long axis of lower incisor to mandibular plane
18	ManBase	Extent of mandibular base (Go-Gn, 2nd measurement)
19	MaxBase	Extent of maxillary base (APMax-PNS)
20	R.asc.	Cd-Go length of ramus (2nd measurement)
21	S-S′	Perpendicular from point S (starting from the SN line) to point S′
22	Pn line	Perpendicular to SeN, drawn from the soft tissue nasion (N) as far as Pal
23	'H' line	Modified Frankfurt horizontal; parallel to the SeN line which bisects the Pn line from N to Pal (Pn/2 – FH/R.asc.)
24	EL	Aesthetic line. Tip of nose – soft tissue pogonion

3 Angular and Linear Measurements

The reference lines enable us to make angular and linear measurements and determine dimensions in the radiograph. The following angles are determined on a routine basis.

3.1 Angles (Fig. 27)

No.	Points of the angle	Definition	Mean value
1	N-S-Ar	Saddle angle	$123° \pm 5°$
2	S-Ar-Go	Articular angle	$143° \pm 6°$
3	Ar-Go-Me	Gonial angle	$128° \pm 7°$
4	Sum	Sum of sella, articular and gonial angles	$394°$
5	Ar-Go-N	Go_1, upper gonial angle	$52°–55°$

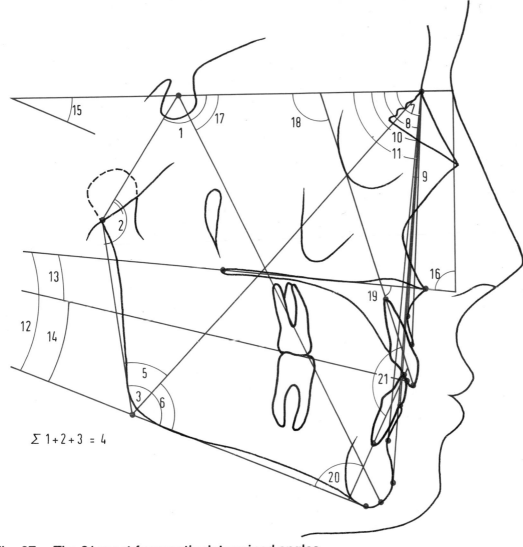

$\Sigma\ 1 + 2 + 3 = 4$

Fig. 27. **The 21 most frequently determined angles.**

6	N-Go-Me	Go₂, lower gonial angle	70°–75°
7	SNA	Anteroposterior position of maxilla	81°
8	SNB	Anteroposterior position of mandible	79°
9	ANB	Difference between SNA and SNB	2°
10	S-N-Pr	Anteroposterior position of alveolar part of premaxilla	84°
11	S-N-Id	Anteroposterior position of alveolar part of mandible	81°
12	Pal-MP	Angle between palatal and mandibular plane	25°
13	Pal-Occ	Upper occlusal plane angle	11°
14	MP-Occ	Lower occlusal plane angle	14°
15	SN-MP	Angle between SN and mandibular plane	32°

16	Pn-Pal	($\angle$ of incl.) Angle of inclincation after A.M. Schwarz	85°
17	N-S-Gn	(Y-axis) Angle between SN line and S-Gn line, anteriorly	66°
18	1-SN	Angle between upper incisor axis and SN line posteriorly	102°
19	1-Pal	Angle between upper incisor axis and palatal plane, anteriorly	70° ± 5°
20	$\bar{1}$-MP	Angle between lower incisor axis and mandibular plane, posteriorly	90° ± 3°
21	ii angle	Interincisal angle between upper and lower central incisor axes, posteriorly	135°

3.2 Linear Measurements (Fig. 28)

28

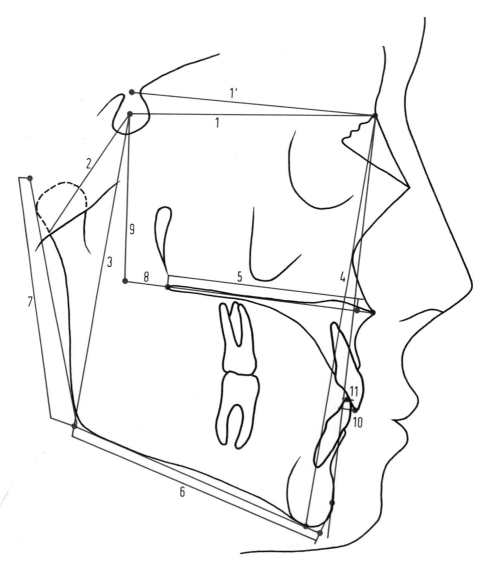

Fig. 28. The principal linear measurements used in the analysis.

We also measure the following linear distances.

No.	Distance	Definition	Mean value
1	S-N	(SeN) Anteroposterior extent of anterior cranial base	71 mm
2	S-Ar	Extent of lateral cranial base	32–35 mm
3	S-Go	Posterior facial height	
4	N-Me	Anterior facial height	
5	MaxBase	Extent of maxillary base, correlated with Se-N (see Table 4, page 62)	
6	ManBase	Extent of mandibular base, correlated with SeN	
7	R.asc.	Extent of ascending ramus, correlated with SeN	
8	S'-F.Ptp.	Distance from S'. to projection of the anterior wall of the pterygopalatinal fossa onto the palatal plane, expression for anteroposterior displacement of the maxillary base	
9	S-S'	Expression for deflections of the maxillary base	42–57 mm
10	1-N-Pog	Distance from incisal edge of 1 to N-Pog line	
11	Ī-N-Pog	Distance from incisal edge of Ī to N-Pog line	

It is not absolutely necessary in practice to use hyphens between the points used to define lines and angles, e.g. N-Pog = NPog, S-N-MeGo = SN-MeGo.

Significance of Angular and Linear Measurements for Dento-Skeletal Analysis

Dento-skeletal analysis in norma lateralis is carried out in three stages:

(1) Analysis of facial skeleton

(2) Analysis of mandibular and maxillary base

(3) Dento-alveolar analysis

1 Analysis of the Facial Skeleton

This consists in determining the saddle, articular and gonial angles, the extent of the cranial base, and facial height.

1.1 Saddle Angle (Fig. 29)

The NS-ar angle is the angle between the anterior and posterior cranial base. Within the region of the posterior cranial base lies a sagittal growth centre, the sphenooccipital synchondrosis. The position of the fossa is determined by growth changes in this area. A large saddle angle indicates a posterior position, a small saddle angle an anterior position of the fossa. If this deviation in position of the fossa is not compensated by the length of the ascending ramus, the facial profile becomes either retrognathic or prognathic. The mean value is 123° ± 5°.

29

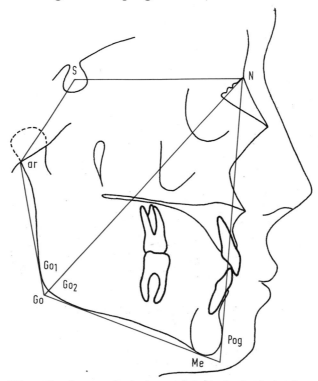

Fig. 29. Sella angle (S), articular angle (ar), gonial angle (go), and upper and lower gonial angles (Go₁ and Go₂).

1.2 Articular Angle (Fig. 29, 30)

The Sar-Go angle is one of those rare angles that may be altered by orthodontics. If the bite is opened by extrusion of the posterior teeth or by distalisation, the angle increases, whilst mesial movement of the teeth will make it smaller. A large articular angle imposes retrognathic changes on the profile, a small angle on the other hand prognathic changes. We have found a reduced articular angle in all cases of prognathism. The mean value is 143° ± 6°.

1.3 Gonial Angle (Fig. 28, 31)

The ar-Go-Me angle is an expression for the form of the mandible, with reference to the relation between body and ramus. The gonial angle also plays a role in growth prognosis. A large angle indicates more of a tendency to posterior rotation of the mandible, with condylar growth directed posteriorly. A small gonial angle on the other hand indicates vertical growth of the condyles, giving a tendency to anterior rotation with growth of the mandible. The mean value is 128° ± 7°. Riolo et al. noted an age-dependent variation in mean value from 132° to 124° (Fig. 32, see page 48).

For accurate analysis, the gonial angle needs to be divided into two, and this may be done in a number of ways.

30

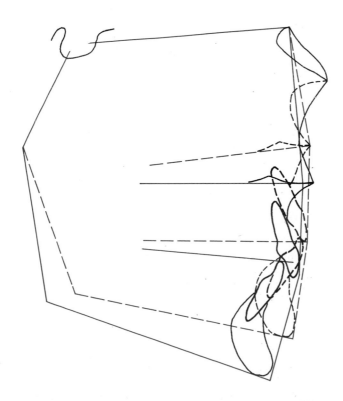

Fig. 30.   A reduction in articular angle may give rise to prognathism. This angle can be changed with orthodontic treatment.

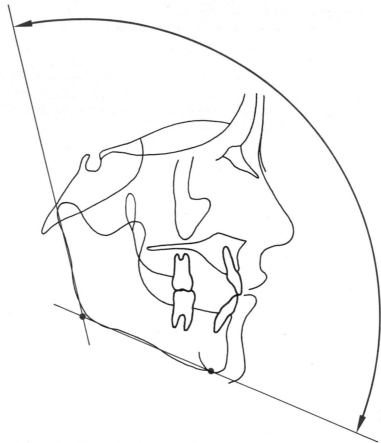

Fig. 31. Gonial angle, determined by articulare, gonion and menton; diagrammatic.

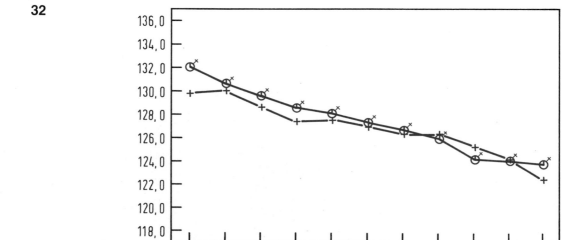

Fig. 32. Age-related changes in gonial angle (Riolo et al).

1.3.1   Upper and Lower Gonial Angles of Jarabak

The gonial angle may be divided by a line drawn from nasion to gonion. This gives an upper and a lower angle (Fig. 29, 33). The upper angle is formed by the ascending ramus and the line joining nasion and gonion. An angle of 50° ± 2° indicates anterior direction of growth. Growth of the ramus leads to prognathism of the lower face in this case. If the upper angle is greater (58–65°), the direction of mandibular growth may be expected to be sagittal, providing the lower angle is smaller (60–70°). If the upper gonial angle is small (43–48°), the direction of growth is likely to be caudal. Generally speaking, a large upper angle suggests horizontal growth changes, whilst a large lower angle indicates vertical growth; a small upper angle relates to caudal, and a small lower angle to sagittal growth.

33

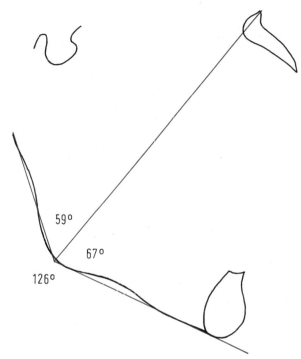

Fig. 33.   Jarabak's upper and lower gonial angles.

1.3.2   Analysis of Mandibular Variations due to Rotation

With the division of the gonial angle we have introduced a further measurement for the following reasons:

The gonial angle has a marked influence on direction of growth, profile changes, and the position of the lower incisors (Fig. 34, see page 50). The magnitude of the gonial angle is determined by the relation between anterior face height and the length of the ramus. Disharmony between these two dimensions will produce extreme variation in the angle. With a relative increase in anterior face height, this angle will tend to be obtuse (as with skeletal open bite), whilst with anterior face height relatively small it is more likely to be acute. On the whole, greater anterior face height is concomitant with a large gonial and also a basal plane angle. The causal relations may vary in such cases:

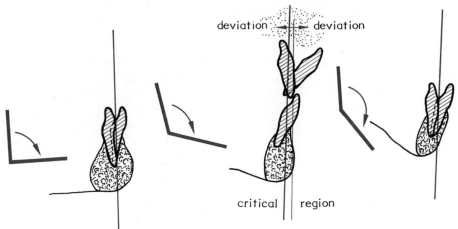

Fig. 34.   Influence of gonial angle on the lower face profile.

(1) The increased gonial angle is due to adaptation to greater anterior face height. Adaptation may also occur in the posterior part of the facial skeleton due to posterior rotation in the temporomandibular joint, with the gonial angle unchanged; the basal plane angle will be increased, however.

(2) The height of the alveolar processes adapts to an a priori large gonial angle, resulting in increased anterior face height.

To analyse these relations in more detail, the following construction was used to relate the gonial angle to the skull as seen in the radiograph (Fig. 35):

A line was drawn at right angles from gonion to the Se-N plane, to divide the gonial angle into a smaller posterior (Go_1) and a greater anterior (Go_2) part. It was assumed that the vertical line thus drawn was the axis for rotation of the mandible. To express this rotation in terms of angles, we examined the correlations between the two parts of the gonial angle and the basal plane angle.

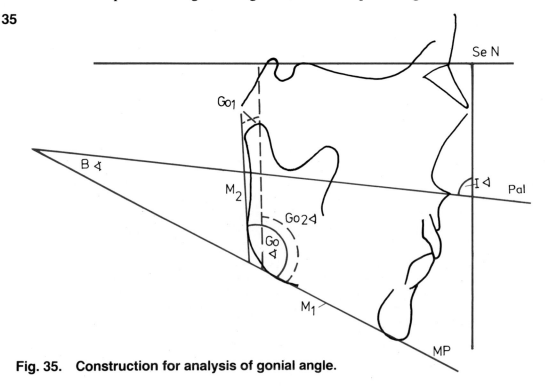

Fig. 35.   Construction for analysis of gonial angle.

1.3.2.1 *Posterior gonial angle (Go₁).* We also determined the range of variation for the posterior angle (Go$_1$) and found that this was considerable. On the basis of Go$_1$, two types of gonial angle could be distinguished:

(1) A gonial angle opening out posteriorly, with Go$_1$ relatively large (Fig. 36);

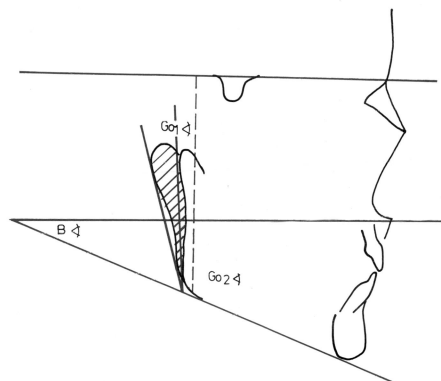

Fig. 36. Gonial angle opened out posteriorly (shaded area).

(2) A gonial angle opening out anteriorly, with Go$_1$ relatively small (Fig. 37).

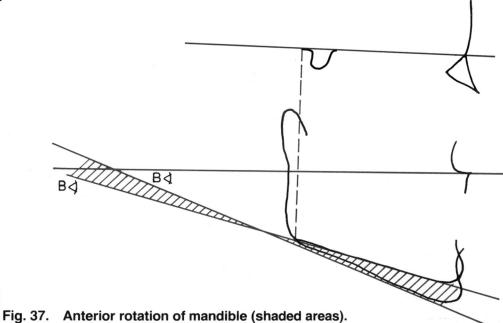

Fig. 37. Anterior rotation of mandible (shaded areas).

In the first type, the basal plane angle (i.e. PAL-MP angle, angle B) was relatively small, in the second, it was relatively large. A positive correlation of Go_1 to PAL-MP angle to facial type was not demonstrable.

There are also cases where the gonial angle is the same, but Go_1 and angle PAL-MP show variations.

A relatively small Go_1 and gonial angle with PAL-MP angle relatively large occurs with forward rotation of the mandible. A large Go_1 angle with relatively small gonial and basal plane angles points to posterior rotation of the mandible. We have analysed the Go_1 angles seen with different types of anomalies (Table 3) and found the mean value to be $5°$, with a range of variation from $-9°$ to $+15°$. Class III malocclusions and open bites had extreme values, despite the fact that the mean gonial angle was almost the same. The reason for this was that open bites very frequently went hand in hand with forward rotation of the mandible (negative Go_1 angles), and prognathism frequently with a gonial angle opening out posteriorly (large Go_1).

Table 3. Go_1 angle with different forms of skeletal anomaly.

Anomaly	Go_1 angle mean	Range	Go angle
Class II_1	$4.5°$	$-3°-12°$	$124°$
Class II_2	$4.8°$	$-1°-13°$	$122°$
Class III	$7.5°$	$-1°-15°$	$130°$
Open bite	$3.9°$	$-9°-14°$	$131°$

1.3.2.2 Anterior gonial angle (Go_1). To eliminate variation due to Go_1, the anterior gonial angle (Go_1) was checked for correlation with the basal plane angle. Considering the anterior angle on its own, the following may be excluded:

(1) Angle PAL-MP becoming smaller in relation to the gonial angle due to posterior rotation of the mandible.

(2) A relative increase in angle PAL-MP due to anterior rotation of the mandible.

(3) A discrepancy between angle PAL-MP and the gonial angle due to the gonial angle opening out to the back, or the ascending ramus tipping forwards.

If the Go_2 angle is used, the posterior side of the angle is standardised (a perpendicular), and Go_2 reflects only variations in the anterior ramus of the angle. Standardisation of the posterior ramus of the angle became necessary when it became apparent, from preliminary studies, that a large gonial angle may be seen also with horizontal growth, if the mandible rotates posteriorly; a small gonial angle may occur with vertical growth types when the mandible rotates anteriorly. By dividing the gonial angle we are able to assess not only the size of the angle, but also its position relative to the cranium, and hence the effect of the gonial angle on the profile. It was found that only the anterior part of the gonial angle (Go_2) has an effect on the basal plane angle; correlation between the two angles was therefore positive ($r = 0.78$).

A correlation of ideal values was established also for angle PAL-MP and Go_2 (with considerable variation, however; Table 4). We were able to determine the relevant angles for the horizontal (first column) and vertical (second column) types of the malocclusions under investigation.

A third, transitional type was found only with Class II malocclusions in the material at our disposal (Table 4).

The ideal values in the table make it easier for us to estimate the type of mandibular growth and express it in angles. At the present time, we do this special analysis of the gonial angle only in problem cases, as a check.

Table 4. Relationship between angles PAL-MP and Go$_2$.

Anomaly	PAL-MP angle	Go$_2$ angle
Class II$_1$	17°–24°	118°–119°
	25°–30°	120°–124°
	31°–40°	125°–134°
Class II$_2$	8°–25°	100°–120°
	26°–29°	121°–130°
Class III	15°–29°	113°–125°
	30°–36°	126°–131°
Open bite	22°–29°	117°–125°
	30°–38°	126°–135°

1.4   Sum of the Posterior Angles (Fig. 38)

The sum of the three above-mentioned angles (saddle, articular and gonial angle) is 396° ± 6° (Bjork). This sum is significant for the interpretation of the analysis.

If it is greater than 396°, the direction of growth is likely to be vertical; if it is smaller than 396°, growth may be expected to be horizontal.

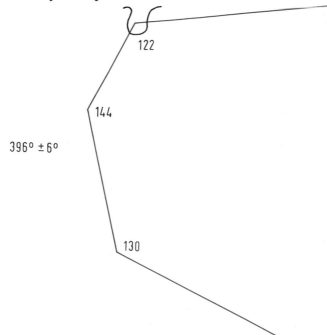

Fig. 38. Bjork's sum of posterior angles (saddle, articular and gonial angle) is 396 ± 6° on average.

1.5 Linear Measurements (Cranial Base and Face Height)

These are done later for technical reasons, in the sequence shown in our case sheet.

2 Analysis of Maxillary and Mandibular Bases

The relative positions of the maxillary and mandibular bases are determined by two groups of angular measurements.

Group 1

Measurements between generally vertical lines, to determine sagittal variation.

Group 2

Measurements between lines that are more or less horizontal, to analyse vertical deviations.

Group 1 consists of measurements of angles between S-N and a third skeletal point in the facial skeleton (Fig. 39).

39

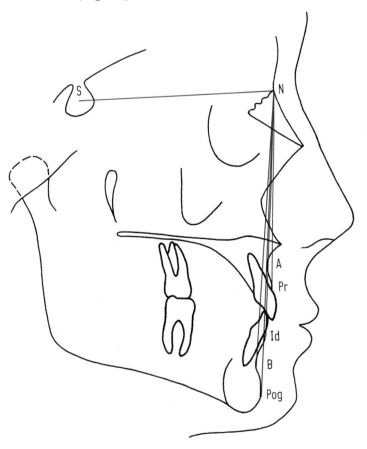

Fig. 39. SNA angle, SNB angle, SN-Pog angle, SN-prosthion and SN-infradentale angles.

2.1 SNA Angle (Fig. 39, 40)

The SNA angle defines the anteroposterior position of point A relative to the anterior cranial base. Its mean value, 81°, indicates a normal relationship between maxilla and anterior cranial base. If the angle is less than normal, the maxilla lies more posterior in relation to the cranial base, if the angle is too large, the maxilla lies more anterior. The angle therefore defines the degree of prognathism for the maxilla. A large SNA angle (greater than 84°) makes the anteroposterior position of the maxilla prognathic, a small angle (less than 78°) makes it retrognathic.

Variations due to age and sex are minimal with this angle (80.5–82°).

2.2 SNB Angle (Fig. 39, 41)

The SNB angle determines the anteroposterior position of the mandible in relation to the anterior cranial base, analogous to the SNA angle for the maxilla. This angle defines prognathism for the mandible, the mean value being 79°. If it is greater than 82°, the mandible is prognathic relative to the anterior cranial base, if it is less than 77°, the mandible is retrognathic. The mandible is described as orthognathic if the angle is between 77° and 82°.

The size of this angle increases with age (from 76° at 6 years to 79° at 16 years of age). Retrognathism may thus be compensated in the course of growth, and it is often difficult to distinguish the effects of therapy from those of growth when Class II anomalies are treated.

40

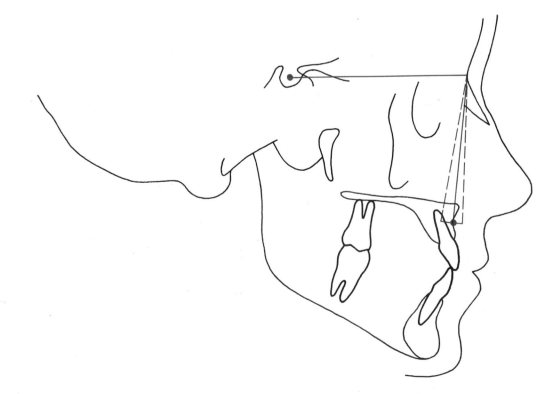

Fig. 40.   SNA angle with range of variation; diagrammatic.

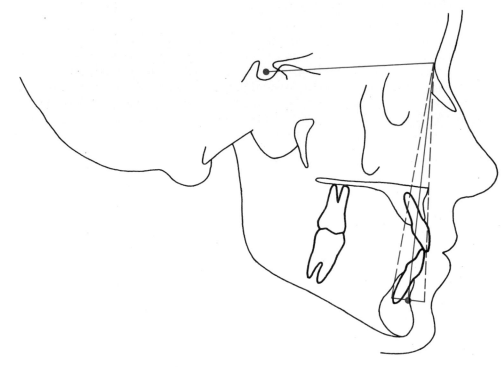

Fig. 41. SNB angle with range of variation; diagrammatic.

2.2.1 Morphology of the Mandible

The three relative positions of the mandible (orthognathic, retrognathic and prognatic) also reflect to some degree the morphology of the mandible (Fig. 42).

2.2.1.1 Morphology of the mandible, *orthognathic* type. Ramus and body are fully developed, with the width of the ascending ramus equal to the height of the body of the mandible, including the alveolar part with the teeth (menton to inferior incision). The occlusal surface runs almost parallel to the plane of the mandible. The condylar and coronoid processes are almost on the same plane, the symphysis is well developed, the lower incisors are almost at a right angle to the plane of the mandible. The SN-MP angle is 18–25°.

42

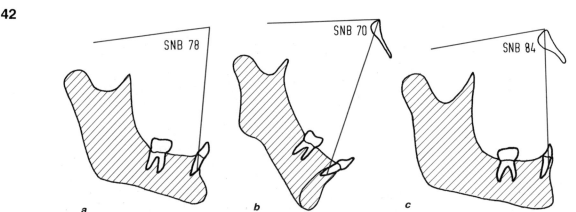

Fig. 42. Variations in mandibular morphology. (a) Orthognathic type, (b) retrognathic type, (c) prognatic type (Jarabak).

2.2.1.2   In the *retrognathic* type, the ascending ramus is narrow, as is the condyle in the anteroposterior direction. The coronoid process is shorter than the condylar process, the mandibular angle is large, the symphysis narrow. The angle between the axis of the lower central incisors and the mandibular plane is greater than 90° (protrusion), whilst the SN-MP angle is 30–40°.

2.2.1.3   In the *prognathic* type, the ascending ramus and the body are wide, the mandibular angle small, the symphysis is well developed. The angle between the axis of the lower incisors and the mandibular plane is less than 90° (very upright incisors), the SN-MP angle is small.

2.3   ANB Angle (Fig. 43)

This represents the difference between the SNA and SNB angles and defines the mutual relationship, in the sagittal plane, of the maxillary and mandibular bases. The ANB angle is positive if point A lies anterior to NB. If NA and NB coincide, the angle will be zero. If, however, point A lies posterior to NB, ANB will be negative. Apart from establishing the relationship between the maxillary and mandibular bases, the angle also largely determines the position of the incisors. On average, the angle is 2°. Riolo et al. found higher averages in children (Fig. 44). High positives occur in Class II, negatives in skeletal Class III.

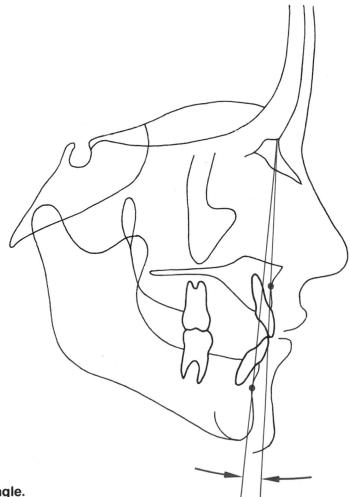

Fig. 43.   ANB angle.

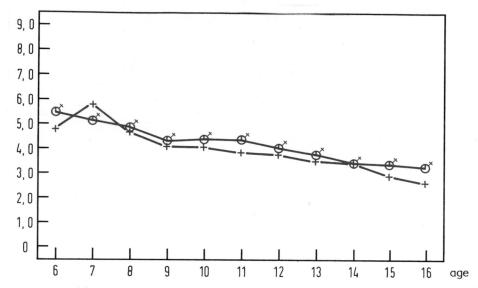

Fig. 44. Age-related changes in ANB angle (Riolo et al).

2.4 Comparison of SNA, SNB and ANB

The three angles referred to above (SNA, SNB and ANB) define the relationship of the maxillary and mandibular bases to the anterior cranial base, and also the mutual relationship of the maxillary and mandibular bases. A number of combinations are possible.

2.4.1 Normal SNA and SNB

This indicates a normal position of the maxillary and mandibular bases relative to the cranial base and also to each other.

2.4.2 Normal SNA

Normal SNA angles indicate normal relations between maxilla and cranial base, with

(a) small SNB angle = mandible retrognathic.

(b) large SNB angle = mandible prognathic.

2.4.3 Normal SNB

Normal SNB angles indicate normal relations between mandible and cranial base, with

(a) small SNA angle = maxilla retrognathic.

(b) large SNA angle = maxilla prognathic.

2.4.4   Both Angles (SNA and SNB) Large or Small

Large angles constitute prognathism of maxillary and mandibular bases; small angles constitute retrognathism of maxillary and mandibular bases.

(a) ANB angle normal: relation of maxillary to mandibular base normal.
(b) ANB angle greater/smaller than normal: abnormal relation of maxilla to mandible.

2.4.5   The 'Wit's' Method

Jacobson described the 'Wit's' (Univ. of Witwatersrand) appraisal of jaw disharmony, which is a measure of the extent to which the jaws are related to each other anteroposteriorly. The method of assessing the extent of jaw disharmony entails drawing perpendiculars on a lateral cephalometric head film tracing from point A and B on the maxilla and mandible respectively, onto the occlusal plane which is drawn through the region of maximum cuspal interdigitation. The points of contact on the occlusal plane from A and B are labelled AO and BO respectively (Fig. 44a). It was found that with normal occlusion, point BO was approximately 1 mm anterior to point AO. In skeletal Class II jaw dysplasias, point BO would be located well behind point AO, whereas in skeletal Class III jaw disharmonies, point BO will be forward of point AO.

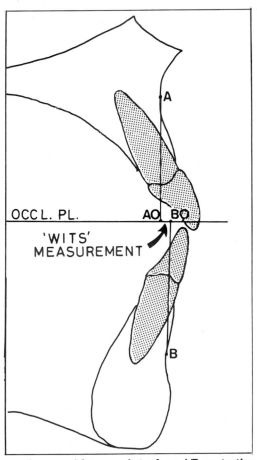

Fig. 44a.   Perpendicular lines dropped from points A and B on to the occlusal plane, Wit's reading is measured from AO to BO.

2.5 SN-Pog (Fig. 39)

The sella-nasion-pogonion angle determines the basal position of the mandible. If the chin projects to a marked degree, the difference between SNB and SN-Pog is large and is 80° from age 16, whilst it is only 76° at age 6, so that one may expect an increase of 4° between age 6 and 16.

2.6 SN-Pr and SN-Id (Fig. 39)

The SN-Prosthion angle defines the relationship between the alveolar processes of the maxilla and the cranial base, the SN-infradentale angle, and the relationship between the alveolar processes of the mandible and the cranial base. These two angles may be used to assess the maxilla and mandible for alveolar prognathism.

These six angles determine relationships primarily in the sagittal plane. They are of major importance for interrelationships in that plane.

2.7 Horizontal Lines

Interrelations within the horizontal plane are assessed to determine the vertical position of the maxillary and mandibular bases. The most important horizontal lines are the SN plane (S-N and Se-N), the Frankfurt horizontal (FH), the palatal plane (Pal) and occlusal plane (Occ), and the mandibular plane (MP) (Fig. 45).

45

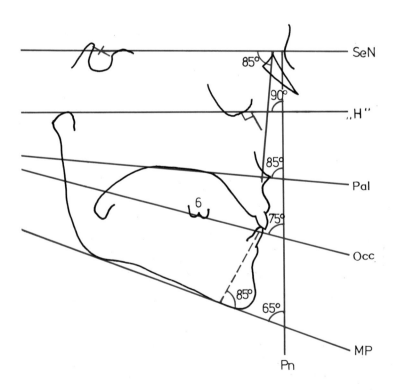

Fig. 45. The most frequently used horizontal lines (A.M. Schwarz).

2.8 Basal Plane Angle Pal-MP (Fig. 46)

This defines the angle of inclination of the mandible to the maxillary base, the latter being represented by the palatal plane. The angle therefore also serves to determine rotation of the mandible. If the basal angle is large, the mandible is usually rotated backwards (vertical growth type), if it is small, the mandible is rotated forwards (horizontal growth type). Our investigations have shown, however, that the size of the basal angle is dependent on the inclination not only of the mandible, but very much also of the maxilla. With retro-inclination of the maxillary base the basal angle will be relatively smaller, with ante-inclination, relatively larger. These changes in the upper side of the angle will change the angle as such, a change not connected with the angle of inclination of the mandible. For a more detailed interpretation of the basal angle, we also measure the inclination, as defined by A.M. Schwarz. The mean basal angle is given as 25°, but there is a very definite decrease in the angle with age, from 30° at 6 years old to 23° at 16.

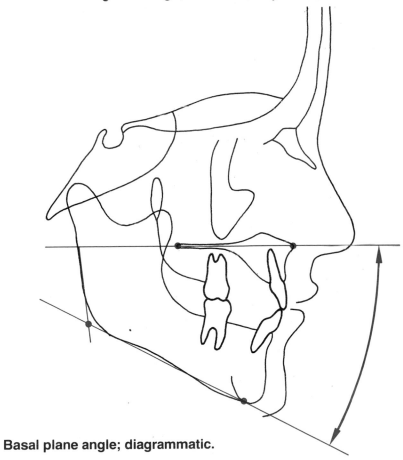

Fig. 46. Basal plane angle; diagrammatic.

2.8.1 Pal-Occ and Occ-MP (Fig. 47)

The basal plane angle is divided in two by the occlusal plane (Occ). The upper angle thus produced (between palatal and occlusal plane) is 11°, the lower angle (between occlusal and mandibular plane) 14° on average. Schudy considered the size of the lower angle important for assessing the prognosis for opening the bite. If the angle is large (more than 20°) the prognosis is good, but if it is small (7° or less) the prognosis is poor for treatment of the deep overbite.

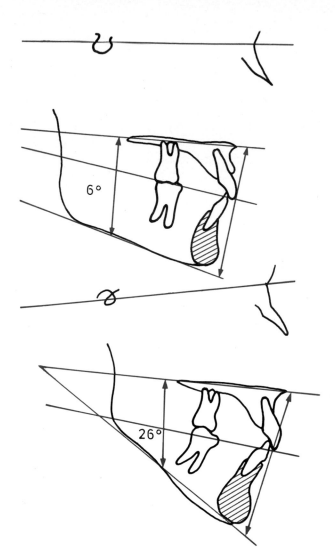

Fig. 47. Upper and lower part of basal plane angle, diagrammatic; (a) small, (b) large angle.

2.9 Angle of Inclination (Fig. 48)

The angle of inclination is the angle between the Pn line (perpendicular from N') and the palatal plane. A large angle signifies ante-inclination, a small angle retro-inclination of the lower face. Determination of the angle of inclination is an absolute precondition for accurate interpretation of the basal plane angle. The angle is also used to assess maxillary rotation (Fig. 49).

2.10 SN-MP (Fig. 50)

This angle gives the inclination of the mandible to the anterior cranial base. Taking the mean value to be 32°, Schudy has introduced the concept of posterior and anterior inclination. If the angle is greater than 32°, inclination is posterior, if less than 32°, anterior. This angle registers vertical dysplasias, changes between sella and fossa and also below the fossa. An open bite, e.g. with an average SN-MP angle, indicates that the molars have come through in disproportion to the incisors.

Condylar and molar growth have been balanced in this case, but were too extensive to achieve a balanced relationship with growth in the region of the frontal teeth.

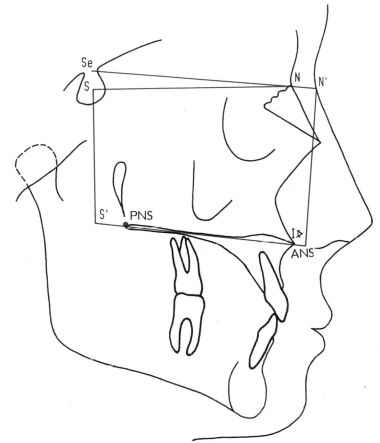

Fig. 48. Angle of inclination (J angle), between Pn line and palatal plane.

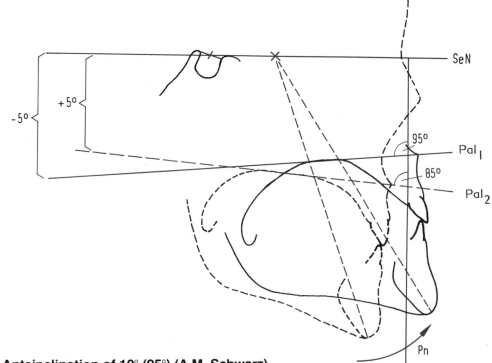

Fig. 49. Anteinclination of 10° (95°) (A.M. Schwarz).

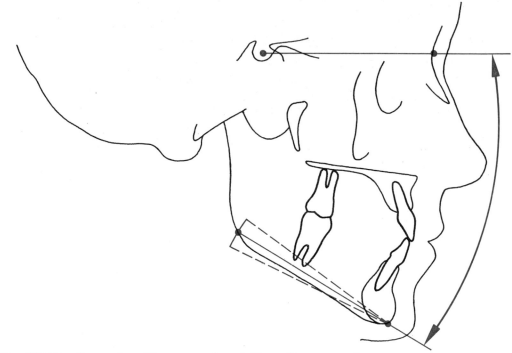

Fig. 50.   SN-Me-Go angle with range of variation; diagrammatic.

If both the SN-MP and the basal plane angle are large, the dysplasia must lie below the fossa (usually the ascending ramus is too short). An age-dependent decrease from 36° to 31° has been noted between the ages of 6 and 16. A vertical dysplasia may be assessed by correlating the four angles we have just been considering. Witt et al. referred to correlation of ANB, SNA and SN-MP, as shown in the following table (Table 5).

Table 5.   According to Witt et al., correlation between the SNA and ANB angle depends on the magnitude of the SNA angle, but also on the vertical relationships (SN-MeGo angle). The tables give the ideal ANB angles for different SNA angles.

SNA<	ANB<	SNA<	ANB<	SNA<	ANB<
68°	1,5°	77°	2,1°	86°	5,7°
69°	1,1°	78°	2,5°	87°	6,1°
70°	0,7°	79°	2,9°	88°	6,5°
71°	0,3°	80°	3,3°	89°	6,9°
72°	0,1°	81°	3,7°	90°	7,3°
73°	0,5°	82°	4,1°	91°	7,7°
74°	0,9°	83°	4,5°	92°	8,1°
75°	1,3°	84°	4,9°	93°	8,5°
76°	1,7°	85°	5,3°	94°	8,9°

2.11 N-S-Gn (Y-Axis) (Fig. 51)

This angle determines the position of the mandible relative to the cranial base, as an additional check. It has a mean value of 66°; if it is greater than that, the mandible is in a posterior position, with growth predominantly vertical. If the angle is less than 66°, the mandible is in an anterior position relative to the cranial base, and growth is predominantly anterior.

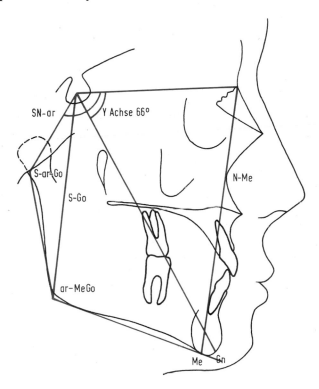

Fig. 51.   Y axis. Anterior and posterior face height largely determine the direction of growth.

2.12 Anterior and Posterior Face Height (Figs. 51, 52, 53)

The next measurement on our record sheet is a linear one. We determine anterior and posterior face height, and use the results to arrive at a figure for the direction of growth. The formula is as follows:

Posterior face height (SGo) × 100: anterior face height (NMe).

The mean value for this is 62–65% (Jarabak). A higher percentage means a relatively greater posterior face height and horizontal growth. A small percentage denotes a relatively shorter posterior face height and vertical growth.

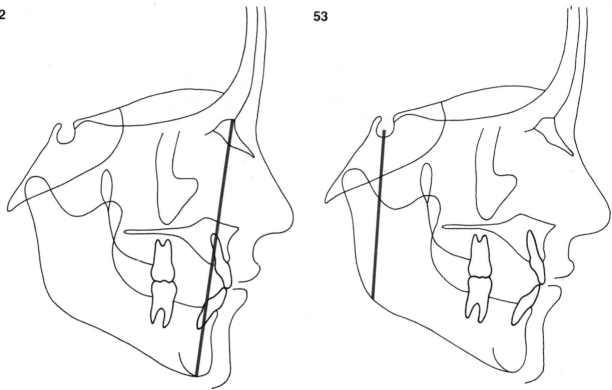

Fig. 52.   Anterior face height.   Fig. 53.   Posterior face height.

3   Dento-alveolar Analysis

This considers the angulation of the incisors, and frequently also of the sixth-year molars.

3.1   Angulation of Upper Incisors

Two determinations are done of the angulation of the upper incisor, its long axis considered in relation firstly to the SN and secondly palatal planes. If the evidence from both determinations is clear, these measurements will permit important conclusions relating to treatment planning, e.g. regarding the need for root torquing. If the evidence is contradictory, it will be necessary to determine which of the two measurements is the more reliable. The inclination of the palatal and the SN plane, the SN-MP and the basal plane angles need also to be taken into consideration.

3.1.1   First Measurement

For the first measurement, the long axis of the upper incisor (Is $\underline{1}$ – Ap $\underline{1}$) is extended to intersect the SN line and the posterior angle is measured. It has a mean of $102° \pm 2°$. Up to the 7th year, it is only $94-100°$ on average, with $102°$ angulation achieved only 1 or 2 years after eruption. Larger angles usually indicate maxillary incisor protrusion, smaller angles very upright incisors (Fig. 54, 55).

3.1.2 Second Measurement

Next, the anterior angle between the long axis of the incisor and the palatal plane is measured. The mean value from the 8th year onward is 70° ± 5° (the posterior angle is frequently measured, and in that case the mean is 110°). An enlarged angle signifies very upright incisors, a smaller than average one incisor protrusion (Fig. 54).

3.2 Angulation of Lower Incisor (Fig. 54)

The posterior angle between the long axis of the incisor (Is $\overline{1}$ —Ap $\overline{1}$) and the mandibular plane (MP) is determined. It has a mean value of 90° ± 3°. From the 6th to the 12th year, the angle increases from 88° to 94°. A wide angle denotes protrusion of mandibular incisors, a smaller than normal angle, very upright incisors. Treatment planning, even for simple forms of treatment, always calls for diagnostic analysis of lower incisor angulation. Without this, it frequently is not possible for example to get the correct design of activator for the lower incisors.

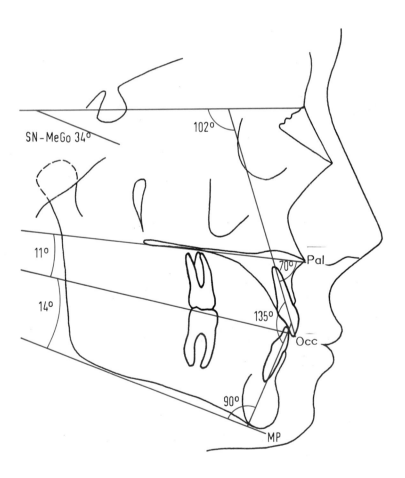

Fig. 54. Measurements to determine angulation of upper incisors (relative to SN and palatal plane) and lower incisors (relative to MP).

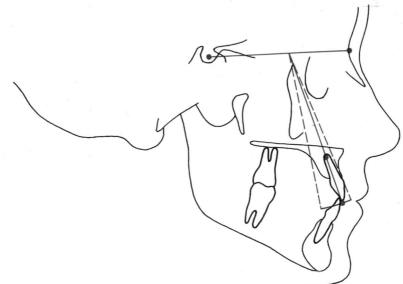

Fig. 55. Angulation of upper incisors relative to SN plane, with range of variation; diagrammatic.

3.3 Assessment of Incisor Position (Fig. 56, 57)

Apart from determining the angles, we also use linear measurements to assess incisor position. The distance of the incisal edges from the NPog line (vertical) is determined. For the maxillary incisor, the average distance is 4 ± 2 mm, for the mandibular incisor, -2 to $+2$ mm. This figure is of considerable importance in treatment planning. The aim of treatment – at least with the permanent dentition – is to achieve those normal relations to the NPog line. This particular measurement (Fig. 58) therefore, is frequently the key factor in deciding:

(a) whether extraction is indicated,

(b) whether the lower incisors can be moved forward,

(c) whether anchorage is critical.

Until the 9th year, these metric relations in the mandible are not sufficiently stabilised to serve as the basis for major diagnostic decisions. In the mixed dentition period, interpretation must consider the phases of active growth still to come.

Riolo et al. have noted considerable age-dependent deviations from normal incisor angulation in the maxilla (Fig. 59). This should be kept in mind for the interpretation of the measurements.

3.4 Inter-incisal Angle

The angle between the long axes of the maxillary and mandibular incisors is also determined. It has a mean value of 135°. A good incisal angle on conclusion of treatment is a major factor in denture stability and prevention of relapse.

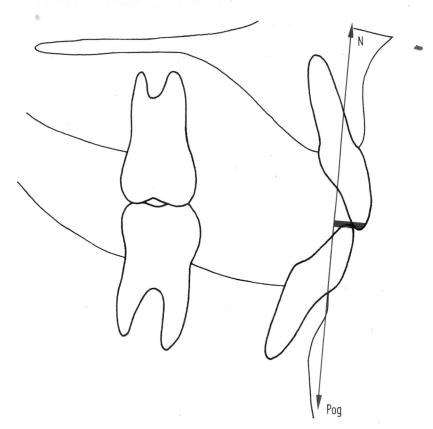

Fig. 56.   Relation of upper incisors to nasion-pogonion plane.

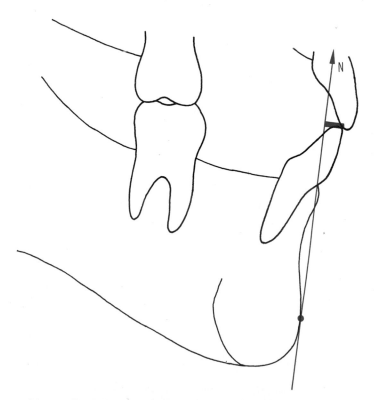

Fig. 57.   Relation of lower incisors to nasion-pogonion plane.

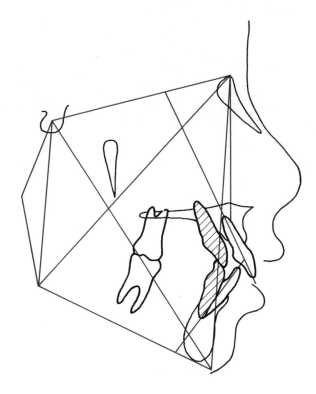

Fig. 58. Consideration of position of incisors relative to nasion-pogonion plane in treatment planning.

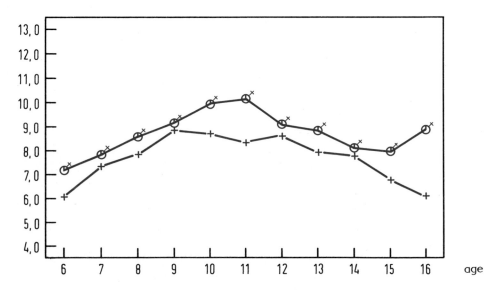

Fig. 59. Age-related changes in position of upper incisors relative to nasion-pogonion plane (Riolo et al).

4 Linear Measurements on Skeletal Structures

We also make a number of linear measurements on the skeletal structures.

4.1 Extent of Anterior Cranial Base, Sella Entrance – Nasion

This distance is used to assess the proportional lengths of the maxillary and mandibular bases. According to Holdaway, it increases by ¾ mm annually. Broadbent and Bolton have determined the mean annual growth rate from age 1 to 18 (Table 6).

Table 6. Changes in extent of anterior cranial base, between the ages of 1 and 18 (Broadbent and Bolton).

	SN line			SN line	
Age	Boys	Girls	Age	Boys	Girls
1	56.3	54.4	10	69.5	66.8
2	59.9	57.9	11	69.8	67.6
3	62.4	59.8	12	70.9	68.4
4	63.6	61.8	13	71.4	69.2
5	65.0	63.4	14	72.3	69.5
6	66.0	63.4	15	73.8	69.7
7	67.2	64.4	16	74.0	69.5
8	68.3	65.2	17	75.1	69.5
9	68.6	65.9	18	75.4	70.1

4.2 Extent of Posterior Cranial Base, Sella – Articulare (Fig. 60)

The extent of the posterior cranial base relates to the position of the mandibular fossa and therefore has a major effect on the profile. A short posterior cranial base denotes a shorter distance between sella and articulare; the mid-face appears more prognathic, with a secondary reduction in anterior face height. The mean value is 32–35 mm, with a mean rate of increase of 8 mm between age 6 and 16.

4.3 Dimensions of Mandibular and Maxillary Base

The dimensions of the mandibular and maxillary bases and of the ascending ramus are assessed in relation to the extent of SeN. We use the measurements proposed by A.M. Schwarz and have compiled a table (Table 7) for the ideal dimensions of mandibular base, maxillary base, and ascending ramus (Fig. 61).

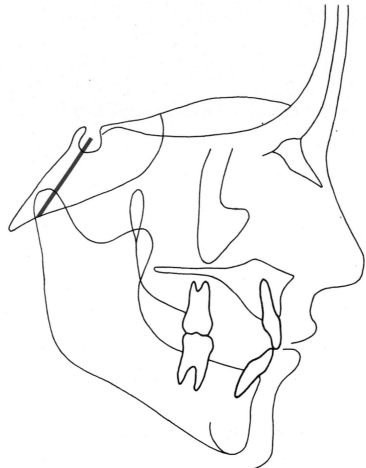

Fig. 60. Extent of posterior cranial base (sella-articulare).

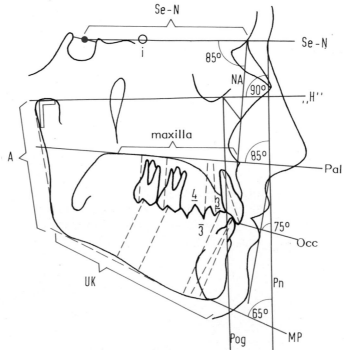

Fig. 61. Analysis of maxillary and mandibular base (A.M. Schwarz).

4.3.1 Extent of Mandibular Base (Fig. 62)

This is determined by measuring the distance gonion – pogonion (projected onto the mandibular plane). The mean value is 68 mm at age 8, with an annual increase of 2 mm for boys and 1.4 mm for girls (up to age 16).

4.3.2 Extent of Maxillary Base (Fig. 63)

This is based on the distance from the posterior nasal spine to point A projected onto the palatal plane. The mean value is 45.5 mm at age 8, with an annual increase of 1.2 mm for boys and 0.8 mm for girls.

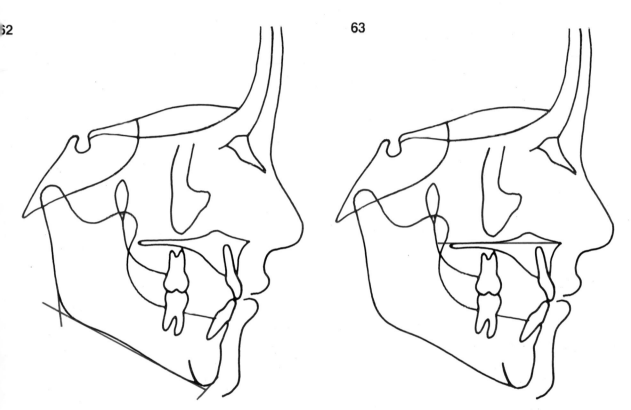

Fig. 62. **Extent of mandibular base.**

Fig. 63. **Extent of maxillary base.**

4.3.3 Extent of Ascending Ramus (Fig. 64)

This is represented by the distance gonion to condylion. Location of condylion may present difficulties, and we therefore construct an ideal Frankfurt horizontal and intersect this with the tangent to the ascending ramus. The point of intersection then represents the constructed condylion.

The ideal Frankfurt horizontal plane is constructed as follows (Fig. 65): The distance between soft tissue nasion and palatal plane, along the Pn line, is bisected. From the point thus obtained a straight line (H line) is drawn parallel to SeN. This represents the ideal Frankfurt horizontal.

The mean for the extent of the ascending ramus at age 8 is 46 mm, with an annual increase of 2 mm for boys and 1.2 mm for girls, up to age 16.

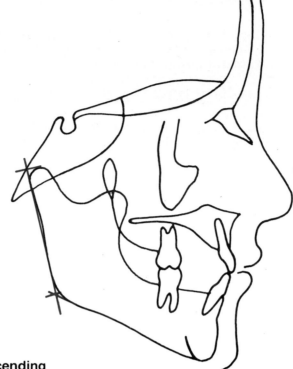

Fig. 64.   Extent of ascending ramus.

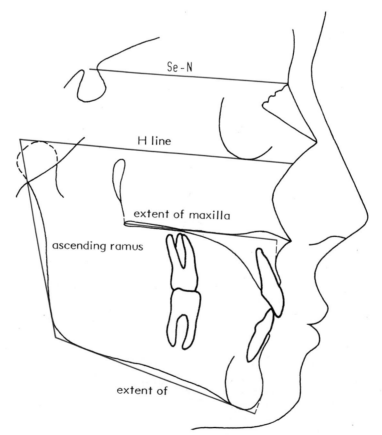

Se - N

H line

extent of maxilla

ascending ramus

extent of

Fig. 65.   Construction of ideal Frankfurt horizontal.

Table 7. Comparative linear measurements of maxillary and mandibular bases and ascending ramus.

Mandible	Maxilla	R.asc.	Ramus	Mandible	Maxilla	R.asc.	Ramus
56	37	40	22	71	47	50.5	28
57	38	40.5	22.5	72	48	51	29
58	39	41	23	73	48.5	52	29
59	39	42	23.5	74	49	53	29.5
60	40	43	24	75	50	53.5	30
61	40.5	43.5	24	76	50.5	54	30
62	41	44	24.5	77	51	55	31
63	42	45	25	78	52	55.5	31
64	42.5	45.5	25.5	79	52.5	56	31.5
65	43	46	26	80	53	57	32
66	44	47	26	81	54	58	32
67	44.5	47.5	27	82	54.5	58.5	32.5
68	45	48	27	83	55	59	33
69	46	49	27.5	84	56	60	33.5
70	46.5	50	28	85	57	60.5	34

Table 8. Multinormative table (according to age) of the principal linear measurements.

Age	N–ANS	ANS–ME	S–N	S–Gn	Ar–Gn
6 yrs	42.5	51.2	64.7	102.6	36.4
8 yrs	45.2	54.2	66.8	108.8	38.8
10 yrs	47.5	56.0	68.2	112.8	39.8
12 yrs	50.0	58.8	69.6	117.5	42.4
13 yrs	50.8	59.8	70.3	120.1	43.8
14 yrs	51.6	61.5	70.9	123.1	45.7
16 yrs	53.2	63.8	71.8	126.8	47.8

Table 9. Multinormative table (according to age) of the principal angular measurements.

Age	SN–Pog	SN–GoGn	SN–Ar	Ar–GoGn	B<	SNA	SNB
6 yrs	78.3	32.4	119.3	129.6	25.6	82.3	78.3
8 yrs	79.2	31.6	120	127.8	24.5	82.1	78.6
10 yrs	80.1	31	120.4	127.2	23.8	82.5	79.2
12 yrs	80.2	31.2	122	127.6	23.3	82.3	79.2
13 yrs	81.3	30.2	121.8	126.4	22.7	83.5	80.2
14 yrs	81.9	29.4	121.8	125.6	22.2	83.9	80.8
16 yrs	82.2	29.4	122.2	125.2	21.6	83.7	80.9

4.3.4 Width of Ascending Ramus (Fig. 66)

This is determined at the height of the occlusal plane. The mean width is 27mm at age 8, and at age 16 is 32.5 mm for boys, 30.5 mm for girls.

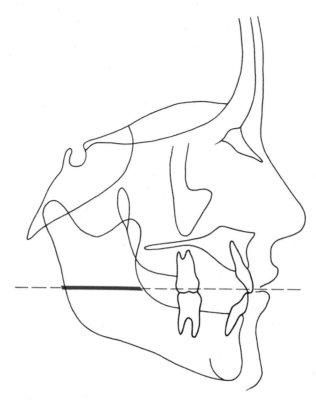

Fig. 66. Width of ascending ramus.

4.4 Assessment of the Position of Maxilla in the Posterior Section

Certain measurements are made to determine the position of the maxilla in the posterior section. A line is drawn at right angles to SN from point S; its intersection with the palatal plane is called S′. The distance from S′ to the posterior nasal spine enables us to assess the position of the maxilla in the horizontal plane. S-S′ on the other hand provides information on vertical relations for the posterior maxillary base (Fig. 67).

Fig. 68 gives a summary of the principal measurements used in analysis. (See also Tables 8 and 9.)

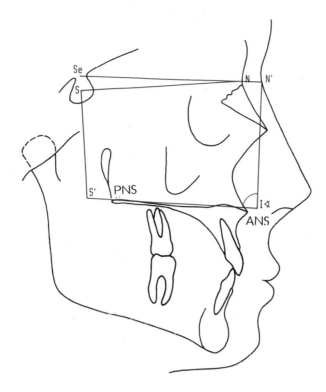

Fig. 67. Vertical and horizontal measurements with the aid of the S-S′ reference line.

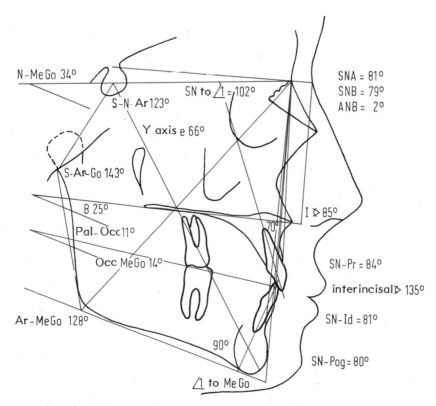

Fig. 68. Diagram showing the principal parameters used in the analysis.

Soft Tissue Analysis

The changes occurring in soft tissue profile in the course of orthodontic therapy represent a major problem. Relatively few techniques or routine methods of soft tissue analysis have been established. One of the reasons why soft tissue analysis has been neglected is that orthodontic therapy was primarily concerned with the correction of hard structures. The results of functional treatment methods and relapses on the one hand, despite satisfactory correction of dentoskeletal morphological relations on the other, have repeatedly and clearly demonstrated the importance of soft tissue morphology. The assumption that soft tissues will automatically adapt to corrected dentoskeletal relations has not been confirmed in practice, as shown in making the aesthetic prognosis. Aesthetic aspects need to be seriously considered, being a factor of prime importance in the motivation of patients coming for treatment.

A good mechanical relationship between mandibular and maxillary dentures was formerly regarded as the sole aim of orthodontic treatment. In the course of time, however, orthodontists have become increasingly aware that facial aesthetics must also be considered in planning.

Angle used terms like balance, harmony, beauty and ugliness in relation to the profile. In 1907 he wrote: "the study of orthodontics is indissolubly bound up with the study of art where the human face is concerned. The mouth is a very decisive factor in determining the beauty and balance of the face." Angle's ideal face was based on the Greek statue known as the Apollo Belvedere. In his opinion, facial aesthetics depended on the position of the upper incisors, a view recently confirmed in the Holdaway analysis. According to Wuerpel, a face is beautiful and shows harmonious features if the proportions of its individual components are right, i.e. no individual structure is over emphasised in relation to the others. This is what he refers to as 'balance'.

For soft tissue analysis, distinction is made between:

(1) Profile analysis.

(2) Lip analysis.

(3) Tongue analysis.

1   Profile Analysis

Case was one of the first to concern himself seriously with profile analysis. He took plaster casts of faces to demonstrate the effects of malocclusions and the results of treatment. In his opinion a balanced profile should be one of the key factors in deciding on the method of treatment for any form of malocclusion.

His assessment of the face is based on the relations between the chin, cheeks, forehead and the dorsum of the nose. In addition he considers the relationship of lips to chin, upper to lower lip, and also the position of the lips at rest, during speech and when laughing.

Soft tissue analyses by cephalometric radiography, using contrast media, have been done by Carrera (1922), McCoven (1923), Comte (1927), A.M. Schwarz (1929) and others. Simpson (1928) produced two radiographs, one hard and one soft. Bjork (1950) placed an aluminium filter in front of the cassette. We also use a filter for soft tissue profiles, and contrast media to outline the tongue.

The standards on which aesthetic assessment is based are:

(a) Classical works of art.

(b) Subjects with perfect occlusion.

(c) Beauty queens, ideals of beauty.

According to Subtelny, every orthodontist has his own concept of an ideal profile that exists in his mind only.

Downs considers that there is a particular average face and profile; faces deviating from the average in particular areas must compensate for this in other structures to present a balanced, harmonious appearance. Extreme deviations cannot be compensated, so that disharmony and imbalance result.

1.1   Reference Points Used in Profile Analysis (Fig. 69)

Profile analysis is based on a number of soft tissue points (indicated by small letters).

Code	Definition
tr	trichion (hairline)
n	skin nasion
no	tip of nose
sn	subnasale
ss	subspinale (concavity of upper lip)
ls	labrale superius (border of upper lip)
sto	stomion (central point of the interlabial gap)
li	labrale inferius (border of lower lip)
sm	submentale (labiomental fold)
pog	skin pogonion
gn	skin gnathion

Two skeletal points are also needed for constructing the reference lines used in profile analysis.

Or	orbitale, a point the width of the palpebral fissure below the pupil
P	porion, highest point on the auditory meatus

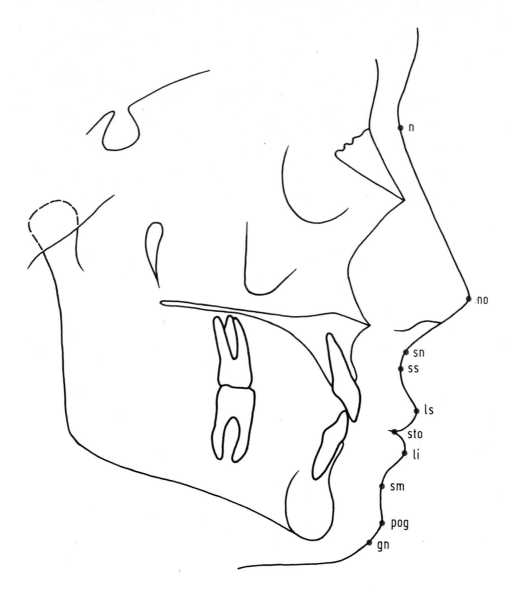

Fig. 69. Soft tissue points for profile analysis.

1.2 Assessment of Total Profile

1.2.1 Proportional Analysis

The search for the profile with ideal proportions is one of the oldest aims of art. These ideal proportions provide the basic standard for assessment of the average profile (mean value, biometric mean, or average). The profile may be divided into three approximately equal parts (Fig. 70):

frontal third	tr-n	⅓
nasal third	n-sn	⅓
gnathic third	sn-gn	⅓

The gnathic third may be up to a tenth greater rather than smaller.

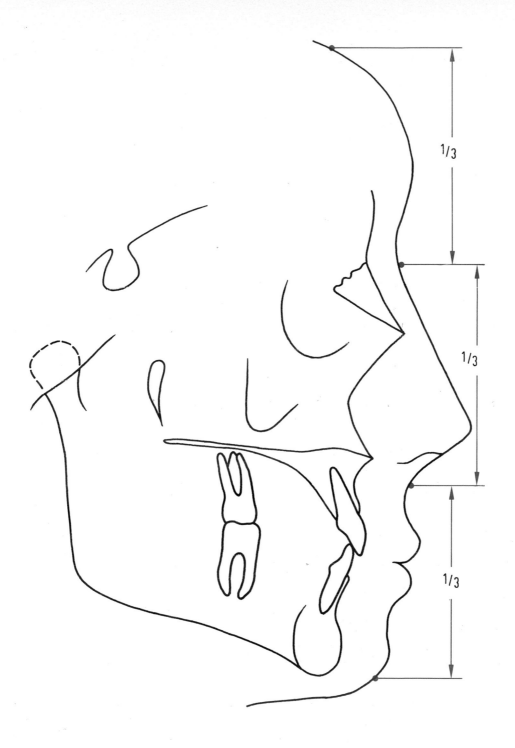

Fig. 70. The division of the profile into thirds.

Similar proportions may be seen with respect to anterior face height, n-gn, with the mid-face (n-sn) occupying 45%, the lower face (sn-gn) 55% of the total height (Fig. 71).

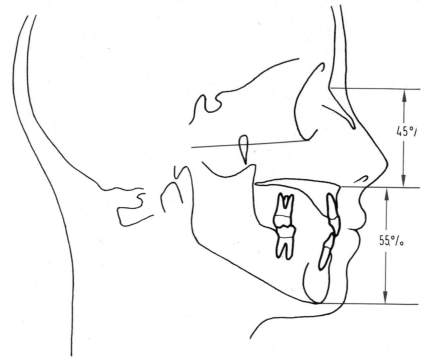

Fig. 71. Proportions of anterior face height (midface to lower face).

1.2.2 Angular Profile Analysis, Convexity of Profile (Fig. 72)

Subtelny makes the distinction between convexity of:

(a) The skeletal profile.

(b) The soft tissue profile.

(c) The full soft tissue profile (including the nose).

1.2.2.1 Skeletal convexity is represented by N-A-Pog, with a mean value of 175°. We have found the mean value at age 12 to be 177.5°. This skeletal convexity decreases with age.

1.2.2.2 Soft tissue convexity is determined as n-sn-pog. The mean value is 161°, and this does not change.

1.2.2.3 Full soft tissue convexity is based on n-no-pog. The mean is 137° for men and 133° for women. We have found 137.5° in boys of 12 and 132.9° in girls. This convexity increases with age. The age-dependent changes in convexity demonstrate that soft tissue changes are not analogous to skeletal profile changes. Increased convexity of the full soft tissue profile may be explained as due to anterior growth of the nose.

Table 10 shows the mean values we have determined for the different forms of malocclusion.

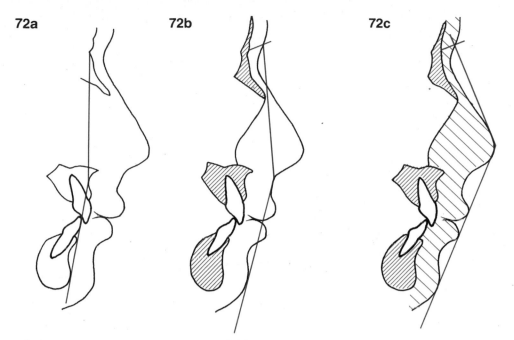

Fig. 72. Subtelny analysis for convexity. (a) Skeletal profile, (b) soft tissue profile, (c) total profile.

Profile	Class I	Class II	Class III
Skeletal profile	174°	178°	181°
Soft tissue profile	159°	163°	168°
Total profile	133°	133°	139°

Table 10. Mean values for convexity.

1.2.3   Thickness of Soft Tissue Profile

Subtelny furthermore determined the thickness of the soft tissue profile and established the following:

(a) The thickness of soft tissue nasion was practically constant.

(b) The thickness at the sulcus lab.sup. increased by approx. 5 mm.

(c) The thickness of the soft tissue chin increased by approx. 2 mm.

In his view, the greater increase in maxillary as distinct from mandibular soft tissue explains why the soft tissue profile grows more convex with age, despite the tendency of the skeletal profile to straighten out.

Burstone gave the following mean values (Table 11, see also Fig. 73).

Bowker and Meredith measured the thickness of soft tissue parts in relation to the N-Pog line in both girls and boys. Their results are shown in Table 12 (see also Fig. 74).

This shows the growth-related changes in soft tissue profile to be expected in the course of treatment.

	Boys	Girls
	mm	mm
Glabella	7	6.6
Subnasale	18.7	16.9
Sulcus lab. sup.	16.2	14.7
Sulcus lab. inf.	12.9	11.6
Soft tissue chin	12.8	12.2

Table 11. Thickness of soft tissue profile (Burstone).

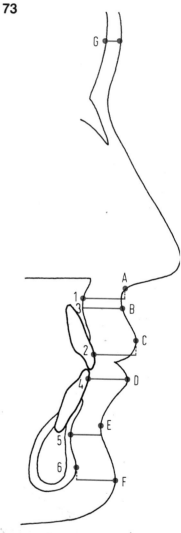

Fig. 73. Burstone analysis. Skeletal points: (1) subspinale, (2) incisio sup., (3) Pro section of point B, (4) incisio inf., (5) supramentale, (6) pogonion. Soft tissue points: (A) subnasale, (B) sulcus labialis sup., (C) labrale sup., (D) labrale inf., (E) sulcus labialis inf., (F) menton, (G) glabella.

		Age 5	Age 14	Gain
		mm	mm	mm
Nasion	B	6.3	6.6	0.3
	G	6.3	7.1	0.8
Tip of nose	B	23.8	30.9	7.7
	G	24.8	32.0	7.5
Convexity of	B	14.5	16.3	1.8
upper lip	G	14.7	17.5	2.8
Labiomental	B	9.7	9.9	0.2
fold	G	9.5	9.5	0.0
Soft tissue	B	11.3	12.3	1.0
pogonion	G	11.4	12.4	1.0

Table 12. Thickness of soft tissue profile (Bowker and Meredith).

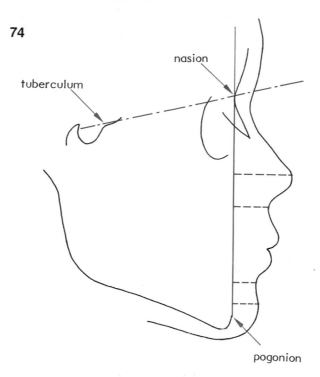

74

tuberculum

nasion

pogonion

Fig. 74. Bowker and Meredith method of determination.

1.2.4 Profile Analysis after A.M. Schwarz (Fig. 75)

Three reference lines are constructed for profile analysis:

(1) The H line, corresponding to the Frankfurt horizontal.

(2) The Pn line, construction of which has already been described.

(3) The Po line (orbital perpendicular), a perpendicular from orbitale to the H line.

The gnathic profile field (GPF or A.M. Schwarz's KPF, for Kieferprofilfeld) permits assessment of the profile. In the average straight face, the subnasale (sn) touches the nasion perpendicular (Pn). The upper lip also touches this line, whilst the lower lip regresses, being approx. ⅓ the width of the gnathic profile posterior to it. The indentation of the lower lip comes close to the posterior third of the gnathic profile field.

The lowest chin point (gnathion) is on the perpendicular from the orbital point, (PO) the most anterior point (pogonion) at a mid-point between the two verticals. The mouth tangent T (sn-pog) is constructed to assess the gnathic profile. It bisects the red of the upper lip and touches the border of the lower lip. With Pn it forms the profile angle (T angle). In the average and all straight faces this is 10°. The width of the gnathic profile field is 13–14 mm in children, and 15–17 mm in adults (Fig. 76).

Depending on the position of subnasale relative to the nasion perpendicular, distinction may be made between the following types (Fig. 77):

(a) *Average face*; subnasale lying on the nasion perpendicular.

(b) *Retroface*; subnasale behind the nasion perpendicular.

(c) *Anteface*; subnasale in front of the nasion perpendicular.

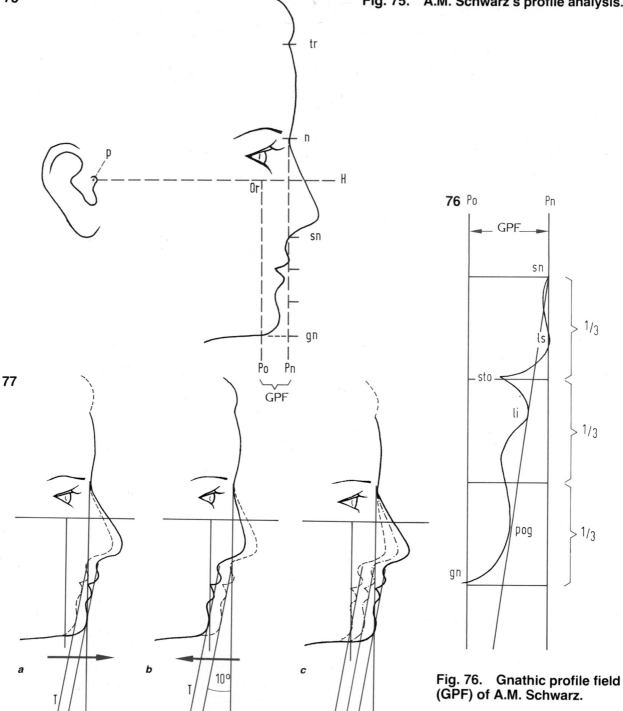

Fig. 75. A.M. Schwarz's profile analysis.

Fig. 76. Gnathic profile field (GPF) of A.M. Schwarz.

Fig. 77. (a) Straight-jawed profile (solid line). The gnathic profile runs parallel and anterior to the average profile (broken line). (b) Straight-jawed retroposition (solid line). The gnathic profile runs parallel and posterior to the mean profile (broken line). (c) The gnathic profiles of straight-jawed anteposition and retroposition run parallel to that of the average face (broken and dotted line), the angle between forehead and nose is more marked with an anteposition and straightened out with a retroposition (after A.M. Schwarz).

If pogonion is displaced proportionately to the subnasale in cases of retro or anteposition, this is known as a straight retroface. This type of straight-jawed face is judged to be as balanced as a straight average face. If pogonion lies more dorsal than normal relative to subnasale, the profile is slanting backwards, if the opposite is the case, it is slanting forward.

The following variations may thus be seen:

1.2.4.1   Three straight profiles:

(a) *Average face.*

(b) *Straight anteface*; the gnathic profile runs parallel and anterior to the average profile.

(c) *Straight retroface;* the gnathic profile runs parallel and posterior to the average profile.

1.2.4.2   Six oblique types (Fig. 78, 79):

(a1) The basic type of oblique *retroface* arises from posterior rotation of the average face; the maxilla is positioned posterior to the average profile, the mandible even more posterior to it (retro-inclination).

(b1) The basic type of *oblique anteface* arises through forward rotation of the average face; the maxilla lies anterior to the average profile, the mandible even more anterior to it (ante-inclination).

(a2) *Average face, gnathic profile slanting backward.* Backward rotation of the profile and posterior displacement of the subnasale are partly compensated by forward displacement of the mid-face, with the result that subnasale is in the average position.

(b2) *Average face, gnathic profile slanting forward.* Forward rotation of the profile is compensated by retrogression in the mid-face area, with the result that subnasale is in the average position.

(a3) *Anteface, gnathic profile slanting backward*, arises through the combined effect of backward rotation and marked forward displacement of the mid-face, bringing subnasale forward of the nasion perpendicular.

(b3) *Retroface, gnathic profile slanting forward.* Combined effect of forward rotation of the profile and backward displacement of subnasale.

1.2.4.3   With a Class II molar relationship (Angle) where the mandible is under-developed, the maxilla being normal, the following relations may be found (Fig. 80):

(a) Average face.

(b) Retroface; one might be deceived into thinking that the maxilla was also underdeveloped.

(c) Anteface; one might be deceived into thinking that the mandible, being in the right position, was normally developed, the maxilla on the other hand over-developed.

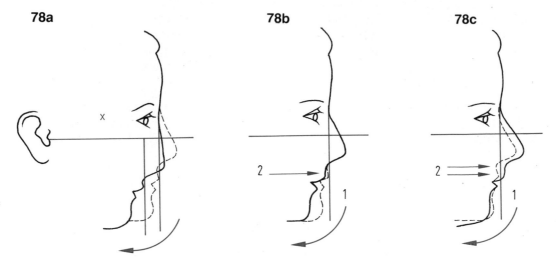

Fig. 78. Three oblique types sloping backwards. (a) Retroposition, gnathic profile sloping backward, (b) average type, gnathic profile sloping backward, (c) anteposition, gnathic profile sloping backward.

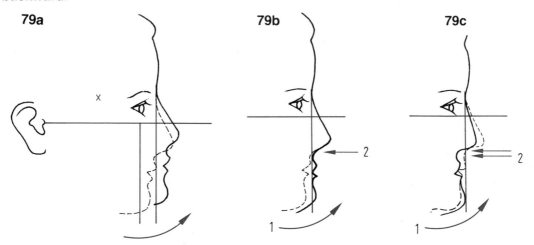

Fig. 79. Oblique types sloping forward. (a) Anteposition with forward slope, (b) average type with forward slope, (c) retroposition with forward slope.

1.2.4.4   With a Class III malocclusion (Angle) combined with an overdeveloped mandible, the maxilla in all cases showing normal development, the following variations may be seen (Fig. 81):

(a) Average face.

(b) Retroface; one might be deceived into thinking that the mandible, being in the normal position, was normally developed, and the maxilla underdeveloped.

(c) With an anteface, it may be wrongly concluded that the maxilla, too, is involved in prognathic overdevelopment.

A.M. Schwarz's profile analysis is of major importance when making an aesthetic prognosis. The aim of treatment is a straight face, for only this will give a balanced profile.

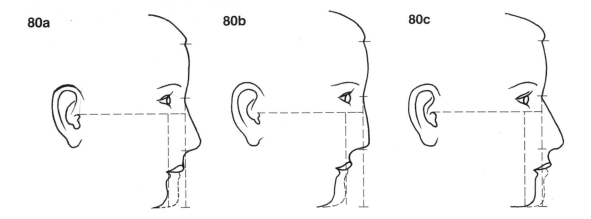

Fig. 80. Angle Class II with mandible underdeveloped, but maxilla normal in all cases. (a) With average type face, (b) with retroposition, (c) with anteposition.

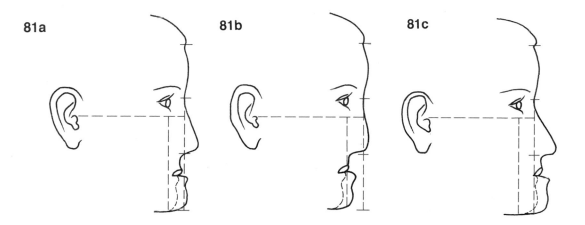

Fig. 81. Class III malocclusion with mandible overdeveloped, but maxilla normal in all cases. (a) With average type face, (b) with retroposition, (c) with anteposition (after A.M. Schwarz).

Certain skeletal factors will influence the profile, chief among them being:

(a) The relative positions of maxillary and mandibular base, i.e. the ANB angle.

(b) Skeletal convexity of the facial skull, i.e. the N-A-Pog angle.

(c) Incisor angulation, i.e. position of the long axes of upper and lower incisors relative to the facial plane (N-Pog).

On the other hand, the soft tissue profile shows changes independent of the bony profile in the following areas:

(a) Nasale.

(b) Infranasale.

(c) Soft tissues of the chin.

2 Lip Analysis

Analysis of the lips plays a significant role in treatment planning.

2.1 Metric Determinations

2.1.1 Length of Upper Lip (sn-sto; Fig. 82)

The mean value given by Burstone is 24 mm for boys and 20 mm for girls. We have found an average of 22.5 mm for boys and 20 mm for girls at age 12.

In Class II (22 mm) and also Class III cases (20.9 mm), the lip is slightly shorter at age 12. A positive correlation exists however between length of upper lip and facial height (N-Gn 104 mm on average with Class II, 101.5 mm with Class III malocclusion).

The upper lip grows only slightly in length with age (between 6 and 12 years), by 1.9 mm on average in Class II cases, and 0.9 mm in Class III cases, slightly more in cases of Class II than with Class III malocclusion.

The upper lip grows longer in the course of treatment, partly due to growth changes, but partly also because of the opening of the bite achieved with treatment (average increase in sn-gn during treatment approx. 3 mm).

2.1.2 Length of Lower Lip (sto-gn; Fig. 83)

According to Burstone, this is 50 mm on average in boys and 46.5 mm in girls; our investigations have shown it to be 45.5 mm in boys and 40 mm in girls.

The lip gradually increases in length with age, slightly more so in cases of Class III malocclusion (with Class II by 1.5 mm on average, with Class III by 1.9 mm on average).

During treatment, the lower lip shows a slightly greater increase in length with mesiocclusion than with distocclusion. The changes are principally connected with growth and increased bite height.

During treatment for Class II malocclusion, following retraction of the upper teeth, the lower lip curls up and moves forward.

During treatment of Class III malocclusion, the lower incisors undergo lingual tipping so that the lower lip moves backwards.

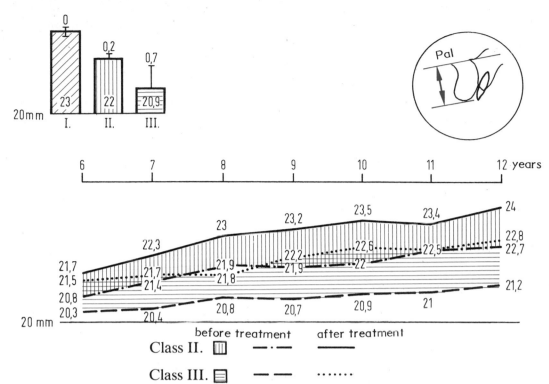

Fig. 82. Length of upper lip with Class II and Class III malocclusion, before and after treatment. Upper left, mean values for Class I, II and III dysgnathia.

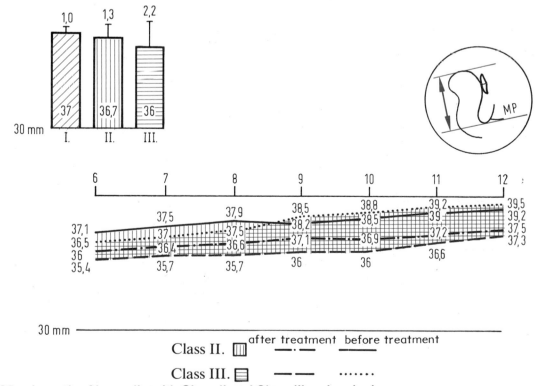

Fig. 83. Length of lower lip with Class II and Class III malocclusion, before and after treatment. Upper left, mean values for Class I, II and III dysgnathia.

2.1.3 Thickness of the Red Part of the Upper Lip (ls-ls; Fig. 84)

This is measured from the labial surface of the most labial incisor to the most anterior point on the red part of the upper lip. The average thickness is 11.5 mm.

With Class II malocclusion, the red upper lip is relatively thin (10.8 mm on average at age 10), with Class III it is thicker (12.4 mm on average). The thinner upper lip seen with Class II is due to the angulation of the upper incisors (63° on average). With Class III the upper lip is also thicker because it rests on a lower lip that has undergone forward displacement.

The upper incisors are retruded during treatment for distocclusion, and protruded during treatment for mesiocclusion.

The thickness increases slightly with age (between ages 6 and 12 by 1.4 mm on average with Class II, and 1.1 mm with Class III). During treatment, the upper lip grows thicker in cases of Class II and thinner in those of Class III, with the result that the difference in upper lip thickness ceases to be significant after treatment. These changes are largely due to changes in angulation of the upper incisors.

The reason is that the upper lip grows thicker as the incisors retract. Following the elimination of lip tension due to 3 mm retraction of the incisors, upper lip thickness increases by 1 mm. Lip tension exists whenever the soft tissue difference between A-sn and the red part of the upper lip is more than ± 1 mm. The lip profile will not change until this tension is eliminated (see also page 106).

Lip tension needs to be considered when assessing the aesthetic prognosis and restoration of lip closure.

2.1.4 Thickness of the Red Part of the Lower Lip (li-li; Fig. 85)

This is measured from the labial surface of the lower incisors to the most anterior point of the red part of the lower lip. The average thickness is 12.5 mm.

With Class II malocclusion, the lower lip is thicker (14 mm on average at age 10), with Class III it is thinner (11.9 mm on average). The thickness of the lip depends on the position of the mandible and on the overjet.

Lower lip thickness increases only minimally from age 6 to 12 (by an average of 1.2 mm in cases of Class II, and 0.8 mm in those of Class III).

In the course of treatment, the lower lip becomes thinner in cases of Class II, and thicker in those of Class III. These changes are due to changes in mandibular position and to pro-inclination of the lower incisors with treatment for Class II, or retro-inclination with treatment for Class III. Retraction of the upper incisors causes the lower lip to curl back or forward. Sublabially, lip contours behave in the same way as the roots of the lower incisors.

2.2 Reference Planes for Lip Profile Assessment

Some authors give special reference planes for lip profile assessment. We use the constructions given by Ricketts, Steiner and Holdaway.

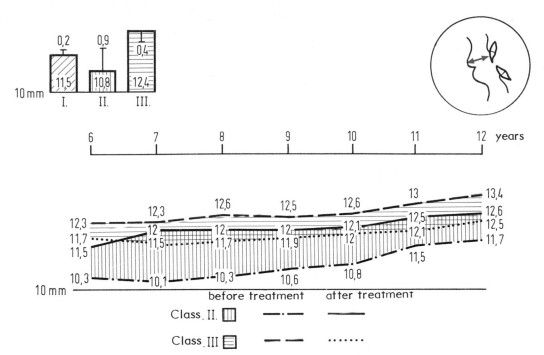

Fig. 84. Thickness of red part of upper lip with Class II and Class III malocclusion, before and after treatment. Upper left, mean values for Class I, II and III dysgnathia.

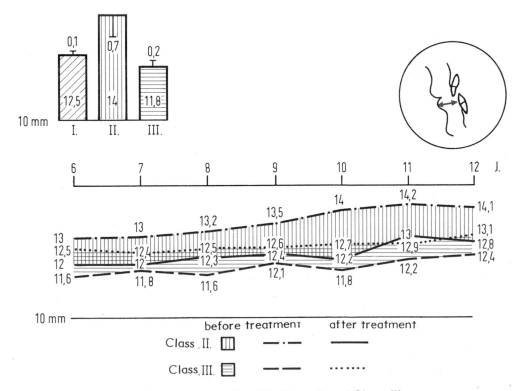

Fig. 85. Thickness of red part of lower lip with Class II and Class III malocclusion, before and after treatment. Upper left, mean values for Class I, II and III dysgnathia.

2.2.1 Ricketts' Lip Analysis (Fig. 86)

The reference line used by Ricketts is drawn from tip of nose to skin pogonion. Normal relations mean that the upper lip is 2–3 mm, the lower lip 1–2 mm behind this line.

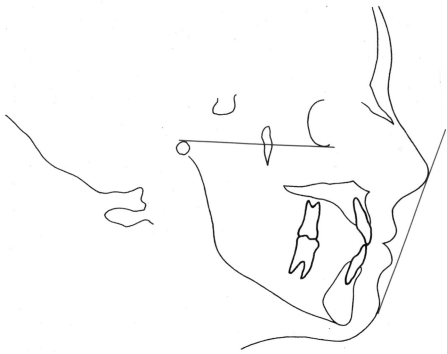

Fig. 86. Ricketts' lip analysis.

2.2.2 Steiner's Lip Analysis (Fig. 87)

The upper reference point for the Steiner analysis is at the centre of the S-shaped curve between tip of nose and subnasale. Soft tissue pogonion represents the lower point. Lips lying behind the line connecting those two points are too flat, those lying anterior to it, too prominent.

2.2.3 Holdaway's Lip Analysis (Fig. 88)

This is a quantitative analysis to assess lip configuration. Holdaway determines the angle between a tangent to the upper lip and the NB line. The angle between these two lines is called the "H angle".

With an ANB angle of 1–3°, the H angle should be 7–8°. Changes in ANB will also mean changes in the ideal H angle (see Table 13).

Holdaway defines the perfect profile as follows:

(a) ANB angle 2°, H angle 7–8°.

(b) Lower lip touching the soft tissue line (the line connecting soft tissue pogonion and upper lip, continued as far as SN).

(c) The relative proportions of nose and upper lip are balanced (soft tissue line bisects the S curve).

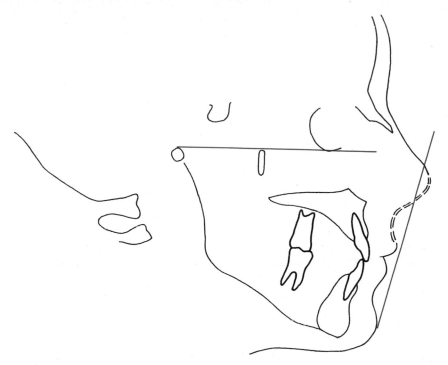

Fig. 87.   Steiner's lip analysis.

(d) The tip of the nose is 9 mm anterior to the soft tissue line (normal at age 13).

(e) There is no lip tension.

The upper lip is tensed if the difference between soft tissue thickness, (A-sn) and the thickness of the red part of the upper lip is greater than ± 1 mm (Holdaway).

Following elimination of lip tension, each 3 mm retraction of the incisors will result in a 1 mm retraction of the upper lip.

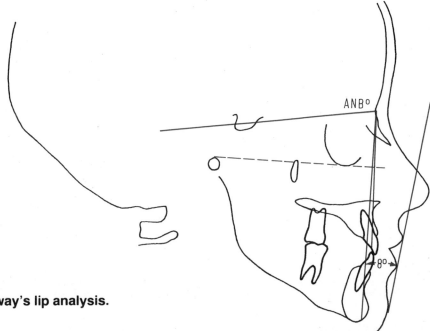

Fig. 88.   Holdaway's lip analysis.

ANB angle	Ideal H angle	ANB angle	Ideal H angle
10°	20°	2°	8°
8°	17°	0°	5°
6°	14°	−2°	2°
4°	11°	−4°	−1°

Table 13. Relationship between ANB and H angle.

3 Analysis of Tongue Position by Cephalometric Radiography

Only a limited number of methods are available for analysis of tongue position in the radiograph. Successful analysis will depend on the right choice of reference line. The preconditions for a reference line that will serve the purpose are as follows:

(1) The greatest possible area of the tongue should lie above the line, as the radiograph cannot show the whole tongue (anatomically).

(2) The line should be independent of variation in skeletal structures.

(3) Its relation to the tongue should not change with changes in position of the mandible.

(4) It should remain constant in relation to changes in tongue position.

(5) It should relate to the anatomical and functional properties of the tongue.

(6) Determination should be as simple as possible.

These requirements can only be met by a line constructed with the aid of a reference point located in the mandible.

Our own determinations are based on the following reference points and lines (Fig. 89):

I = incisal edge of lower central incisors; M = cervical, distal third of the last erupted molar; V = most caudal point on the shadow of the soft palate, or its projection onto the reference line. I and M_c are connected and the connecting line continued to V; this is the reference line. It offers the following advantages:

(a) A relatively large part of the tongue as seen in the radiograph lies cranial to it.

(b) The line is independent of skeletal relationships.

(c) It is independent of changes in tongue position.

The line connecting I and V is then bisected, the point of bisection being point 0. From this, a perpendicular line is drawn to the roof of the mouth.

A transparent template (Fig. 90) is used for the determinations. This has a horizontal line which is placed to coincide with the reference line traced on the radiograph, and a vertical line which should coincide with the vertical reference line. From point 0 on the template, where three lines now meet, we draw four more lines, all at 30° angles. This gives a total of 7 lines, and these are marked out in millimetres. The template is placed on the radiograph and the measurements required for the analysis of tongue position can then be read off.

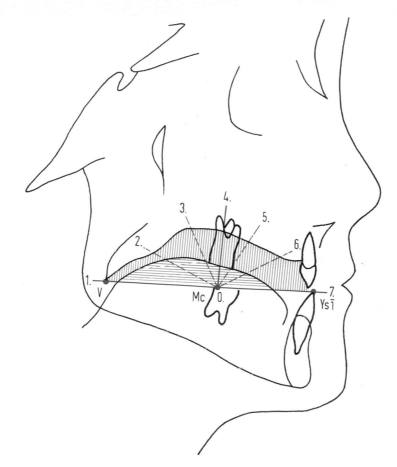

Fig. 89. Construction for assessment of tongue position in the radiograph.

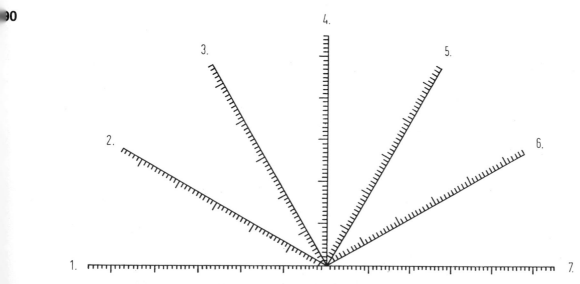

Fig. 90. Template for assessment of tongue position in the radiograph.

3.1 Tongue Parameters

Using the template two types of determination may be executed:

3.1.1 Assessment of Tongue Position

On the radiograph taken in occlusion, the space between tongue and roof of mouth is defined by distances in millimetres (vertical shading in Fig. 89). If the lines on the template are numbered from 1 to 7, the measurement made along 1 gives the distance between the soft palate and the root of the tongue (posterior border of oral cavity), those along lines 2–6 give the relationship of the dorsum of the tongue to the roof of the mouth, and that along No. 7 the position of the tip of the tongue (or its projection onto the line) relative to the lower incisors.

3.1.2 Assessment of Tongue Motility

The second determination relates to the motility of the tongue. For this, the position of the tongue in dental occlusion is compared with that in rest position. The template is used to determine the height of the dorsum of the tongue on all seven lines, in both radiographs (horizontal shading in Fig. 89). The difference between occlusal and rest position is then calculated. This method permits assessment of the actual change in tongue position, independent of the inter-occlusal space. The occlusal position is taken as zero, with changes in position given in positive and negative figures, i.e. a positive figure indicates that the tongue is higher in rest position than in occlusal position, and vice versa.

3.2 Average Findings

3.2.1 Results of Tongue Position Assessment

The results are shown in Table 14.

3.2.1.1 The *root of the tongue* (measurement No. 1). With anomalies in nasal breathing, a small space is found between the root of the tongue and the soft palate (0.9 to 2.1 mm on average). A space in this segment is not always due to mouth breathing, but may also occur with a small tongue (in cases of deep overbite). A small tongue may sometimes also be seen with Class III malocclusion, but it is then in an anterior position, so that the space between the root of the tongue and the soft palate is large. In cases of mouth breathing, the space is also large (5.1 to 5.2 mm on average).

3.2.1.2 The *dorsum of the tongue* (measurements No. 2 to 6) is relatively high with Class II malocclusions. In cases of deep overbite, the dorsum is high at the back, low in front. In all other cases the dorsum tends to be low.

Malocclusion	Measurements in mm						
	1	2	3	4	5	6	7
Class II₁	0.9	3.1	5.0	5.8	7.8	9.1	6.2
Class II₁ with mouth breathing	5.1	8.3	10.2	11.7	12.3	12.2	10.0
Class II₂	2.1	3.7	3.7	7.5	9.4	10.4	8.6
Class III	1.1	5.9	10.2	10.3	10.9	9.8	6.3
Class III with mouth breathing	5.2	9.2	11.6	12.3	11.6	8.4	5.2
Open bite	1.9	5.7	8.5	8.8	11.2	9.2	2.4

Table 14.   Assessment of tongue position.

3.2.1.3   The *tip of the tongue* (measurement No. 7) is retracted in cases of Class III and in Class II cases with nasal breathing (6.3 mm), and even more so in cases of deep overbite. With Class II and mouth breathing the tip of the tongue is considerably retracted (10.0 mm), whereas retraction is less (5.2 mm) with Class III and mouth breathing. In cases of open bite the tip of the tongue lies forward (2.4 mm).

The results are shown in graph form, with the mean values drawn as curves and the two mean deviations in each case as areas. Space permits only one graph to be shown. This compares the tongue positions for Class II and Class III malocclusions. With Class III, we frequently see a lower tongue profile (Fig. 91).

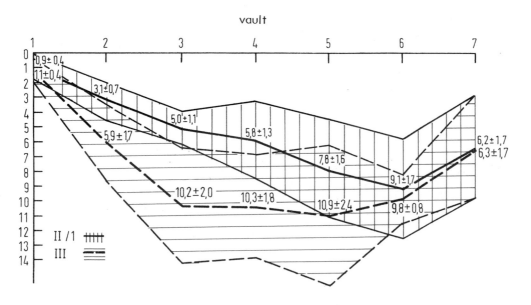

Fig. 91.   Analysis of tongue position in cases of Class II and Class III dysgnathia.

3.2.2 Results of Tongue Motility Assessment

The results of investigations based on comparison between rest and occlusal position of the tongue are summarised in Table 15.

Malocclusion	Measurements in mm						
	1	2	3	4	5	6	7
Class II$_1$	0.4	1.2	−0.8	0.4	−1.9	−2.2	−3.2
Class II$_1$ with mouth breathing	0.3	0.7	0.1	0.0	−0.1	−0.8	−0.3
Class II$_2$	0.2	0.0	−1.4	0.0	−1.2	0.0	0.9
Class III	0.6	1.3	0.8	−0.4	0.1	0.5	3.2
Class III with mouth breathing	−1.4	−1.5	0.1	0.4	0.1	0.2	2.6
Open bite	0.5	0.5	−0.2	−0.9	0.1	−0.2	0.8

Table 15.   Assessment of tongue motility.

Changes in tongue position are predominantly reflected by the position of the tip of the tongue. The position of other parts of the tongue does also change, though not relative to the mandible, but in conjunction with it. The changes in position of the tip relate closely to the different types of malocclusion. With Class II, the tongue is further back in rest position, with Class III it lies further forward. It may be assumed that the changes in position of the tip of the tongue relate to the tendency to mandibular malformation.

Comparison of Class II and Class III malocclusions will show, for example, that in rest position the tip is retracted in cases of Class II, but shows forward displacement in those of Class III (Fig. 92).

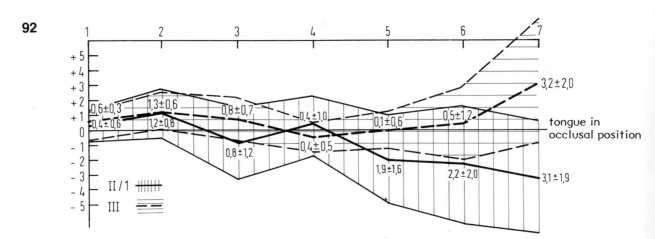

Fig. 92.   Analysis of tongue motility in cases of Class II and Class III dysgnathia.

100

4   Functional Analysis of the Radiograph

Cephalometric radiography will also demonstrate the relationship between rest and occlusal positions. Relative to its occlusal position, the mandible may be further back or further forward than in rest position.

If a radiograph is taken in rest position and another in occlusion, mutual relations between these two may be established. In every movement of the mandible we can differentiate between a rotatory and a gliding component. The principle of comparative assessment consists in the determination of one angle for the rotational component and another for the gliding component (Fig. 93).

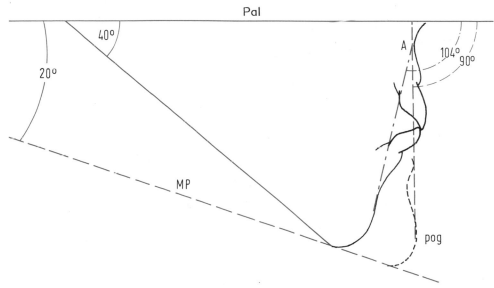

Fig. 93.   Angle B gives the rotational component and angle MM the gliding component for movement from rest to occlusion.

Correlative assessment of the angles at rest and in occlusion will give us the 'differential' values.

The basal plane angle (B angle) for instance can be used to show rotatory movement, and the maxillomandibular (MM) angle (the angle between AB and palatal plane) for gliding motion. The difference between the angles in resting position and in occlusion is represented by the angle B_u for the rotatory component, and the angle MM_u for the gliding component of movement from rest to occlusion (Fig. 94).

We have subjected these relations to statistical analysis and compiled a table of ideal values for Class II and Class III malocclusions with balanced functional relationships (Fig. 95, 96).

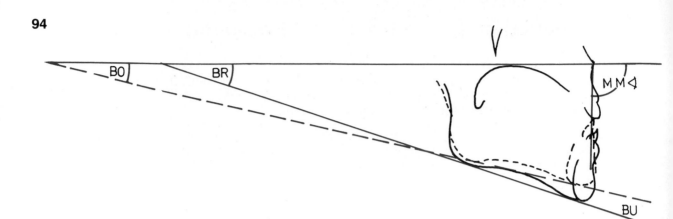

Fig. 94. Measurement of angle B in the rest position (BR) and in occlusal position (BO) serves to determine the differential angle BU.

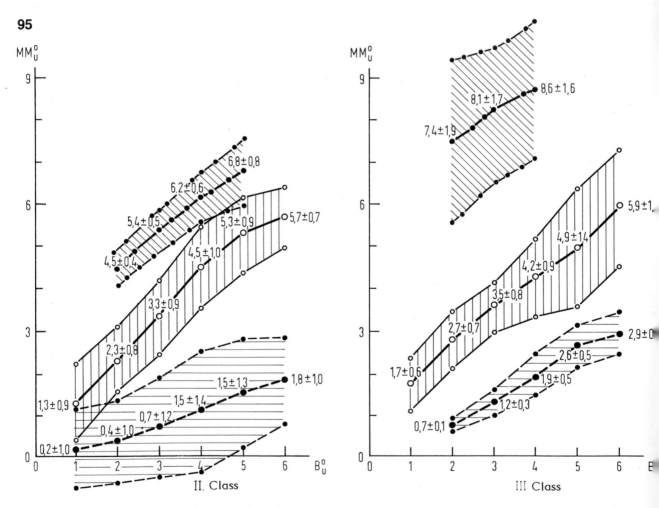

Fig. 95. Graphic representation of the relationship between Bu and MMu in Class II and Class III cases. The middle lines give the mean values. Shaded areas for sigma values, with 'corresponding' cases at the centre, those with backward gliding motion above, and those with forward gliding motion below.

	B_U°	(a) Corres. to average		(b) Backward gliding motion		(c) Forward gliding motion		(d) t_i values between	
								(a) (b) p%	(a) (c) p%
		m_i	σ_i	m_i	σ_i	m_i	σ_i		
Angle Class II	1°	1.16±0.36		—		0.25±1.07		—	<5
	2°	2.62±0.48		4.33±0.46		0.30±0.88		<0.1	<0.1
	3°	2.83±1.10		—		0.70±1.18		—	<0.1
	4°	5.00±1.02		6.40±0.49		1.22±1.90		<2.5	<0.1
	5°	5.11±0.93		6.66±0.93		—		<2.5	—
	6°	5.30±0.75		—		1.85±0.83		—	<0.1
Angle Class III	1°	1.66±0.47		—		—		—	—
	2°	2.71±0.84		7.20±1.88		1.00±0.0		<0.1	—
	3°	3.60±0.48		8.33±1.55		—		<0.1	—
	4°	4.12±0.78		8.44±1.61		1.33±0.47		<0.1	<0.1
	5°	4.66±1.76		—		3.00±0.0		—	—
	6°	6.00±1.00		—		2.66±0.47		—	<0.1

Fig. 96.   The same relationships as shown in graphic representation, in tabular form for Class II and Class III dysgnathia.

Interpretation of Measurements

Determination of the various dimensions in the radiograph is a routine task that may be delegated or done semi-automatically (digitiser 'computer'). The actual medical work consists in interpreting the results.

In the introduction, reference was made to the fact that there are a number of methods of interpretation, the most widely known and used being correlative analysis. The aims of interpretation may be summarised as follows:

(1) To determine the skeletal structure and the facial type.

(2) To establish the relationship between maxillary and mandibular base and determine the type of growth.

(3) To assess dental relationships.

(4) To analyse the soft tissues regarding ætiology and prognosis.

(5) To establish the location of the malocclusion within the facial skull, on the basis of the above analyses, and determine the extent to which it is skeletal on the one hand and dento-alveolar on the other.

(6) Treatment planning – after synthesis of the analytical results – calls for determination of the possible methods of treatment. The question has to be answered, for instance, as to how far treatment can be causal and how far merely compensatory (for skeletal abnormalities).

In the following pages the problems of cephalometric radiography are considered, but it should be emphasised that it is only one of the investigations on which overall case management is based. All investigations need to be considered together before a definite plan is decided upon. Radiographic analysis cannot take the place of clinical diagnosis, and one should not expect a radiograph to provide all the information needed for treatment planning.

1 Facial Profiles and Skeletal Analyses

Depending on the criteria, classification and purpose of the investigation, distinction may be made between a number of facial types. In assessing the relationship of facial skeleton to cranial base, for example, an orthognathic, retrognathic and prognathic facial type may be defined. Cephalometric radiography will give an accurate definition of facial type. No close correlation exists between facial type and anomaly as defined in the present context. A particular facial type may occur in conjunction with different malocclusions or with normal occlusion. On the other hand the same dento-alveolar deviations are frequently seen with different facial types. A statistically significant incidence does however exist for certain forms of malocclusions, such as Class II in retrognathic faces, and Class III with prognathic types of facial skeleton, whilst an orthognathic facial skeleton is no guarantee of normal occlusion.

Individual measurements are of no practical significance when seen in isolation. A normal gonial angle, for instance, does not necessarily mean normal dentition, whilst a large gonial angle need not always go hand in hand with malocclusion.

The facial skeleton has a number of morphological components. Individual components may deviate from the norm, but in combination with the others compensation may well have resulted in normal occlusion. On the other hand individual components may be more or less within normal range, yet an unfortunate combination of components may have produced a malocclusion.

Determination of skeletal relationship to the facial type is important in treatment planning, despite the fact that no definite correlation has been established. With Class II and a retrognathic facial type, for example, treatment will be more difficult and the prognosis less certain than with Class II malocclusion occurring in a face of the orthognathic type. In the same way the prognosis is very much more uncertain when treating Class III occurring with prognathic than with orthognathic or retrognathic facial types.

The anchorage mechanisms, the planning of extractions and many other therapeutic problems will be different with a retrognathic facial type than with a prognathic one.

The facial type also has a considerable influence on dental relationships. Thus a Class II anomaly will usually be dento-alveolar in the orthognathic type with distocclusion, and treatment must be limited to the dento-alveolar region. If the facial type is retrognathic with a Class II malocclusion, i.e. the anomaly is due also to unfavourable skeletal relationships, treatment becomes much more of a problem, the prognosis is less certain, and it may often be necessary to effect dento-alveolar compensation for the skeletal abnormalities.

Skeletal analysis and determination of the facial type is also important for the ætiological assessment of anomalies. With an open bite that can be localised in the dento-alveolar region, for example, the cause of the anomaly is an oro-facial dysfunction. With skeletal open bite occurring with a large basal plane angle and growth related posterior rotation of the mandible (vertical growth type), the dysfunction is usually secondary, and treatment much more difficult, requiring different methods.

1.1 Orthognathic Skeletal Relationship

In the orthognathic face, the maxillary and mandibular bases show normal relationship to the anterior cranial base (SN plane). The SNA and SNB angles are normal. This group usually presents with anomalies involving dento-alveolar abnormalities and a Class I relationship (Fig. 97a, b, 98).

1.1.1 Crowding

With this type of face, crowding is due to discrepancies between the size of the teeth and their apical base or to dysfunction; crowding may be primary (transversal deviation in the frontal plane) or secondary (mesiodistal). For differential diagnosis, it is important to know that with primary crowding the incisors will tend to persist in the bud stage (Fig. 99). With secondary crowding, the position of the incisors is generally normal.

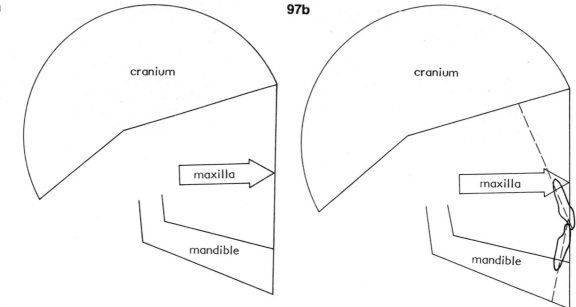

Fig. 97. Orthognathic relationship of facial bones. (a) Relationship of maxillary and mandibular base, (b) dento-alveolar relationship.

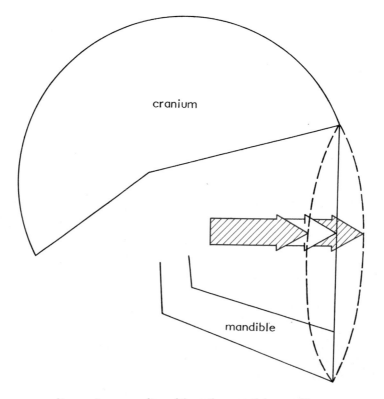

Fig. 98. Midface concavity and convexity with orthognathic profile.

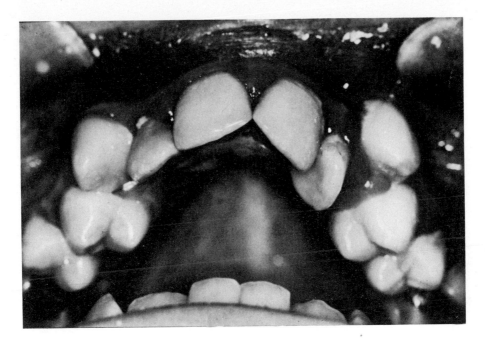

Fig. 99. Bud stage persisting with crowding in the maxilla; palatinal position of lateral incisors and labial position of canines.

1.1.2   Spaces in the Dentition

Spaces in the dentition (gaps between the teeth) are also frequently found with the orthognathic type of face, and these are again caused by a discrepancy between tooth size and dental arch size. Spacing may also occur with incisor protrusion in the upper jaw, the result of dysfunction.

1.1.3   Class II Malocclusion

Relatively frequent with this type of face are:

(a) Distocclusion, i.e. dento-alveolar Class II occlusion with balanced skeletal structure of the face (Fig. 100a, b).

(b) Cases of translocated closure where the mandibular base is well developed, the sum of posterior angles normal, and a normal relationship exists between the jaws in rest position, but there is dental distal translocation in occlusion.

(c) Class II_2 malocclusion, with maxillary and mandibular base well developed, and incisal distal translocation.

1.1.4   Class III Malocclusion

Class III cases may also be seen in orthognathic types, and these are cases of translocation. Differential diagnosis depends chiefly on assessing the extent of the mandibular base in relation to the anterior cranial base, the saddle, articular and gonial angles, as well as functional analysis (see page 126).

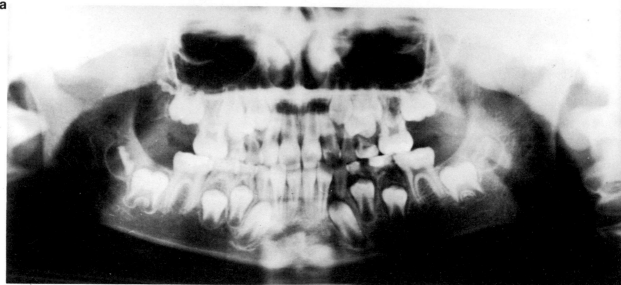

100a

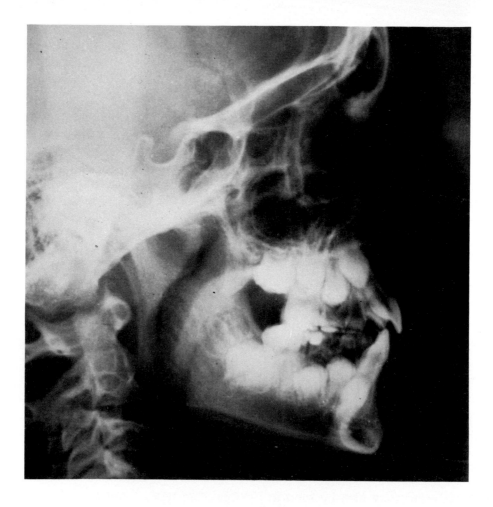

100b

Fig. 100.   Mesial movement of upper 6th-year molars in an orthognathic face. This is a case of distoclusion. (a) Orthopantomogram,
(b) teleradiograph.

1.2 Retrognathic Skeletal Relationship (Fig. 101)

With the retrognathic facial profile, the maxillary and mandibular bases lie posterior to the cranial base, and the molar relationship tends to be Class II. Five types may be distinguished.

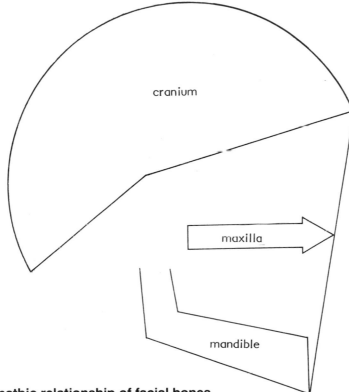

Fig. 101. Retrognathic relationship of facial bones.

1.2.1 Normal Interrelationship of Apical Bases, Class II Malocclusion

In addition to a retrognathic facial structure, Class II malocclusion is in this case usually caused by mesial migration of molars (due to early loss of primary teeth) or by dysfunction. Retrognathia is not very marked, and dento-alveolar Class II malocclusion predominates (Fig. 102).

1.2.2 Anterior Position of Nasomaxillary Complex

The SNA angle is too large, the SNB angle within normal range (Fig. 103).

This type of anomaly is frequently hereditary, with dysfunction also playing a role in the ætiology. This really is a Class II relationship, with the 'fault in the maxilla'. Anterior displacement may be:

1.2.2.1 *Basal*, not involving incisor protrusion, and treatment will have to consist in 'bodily' retraction of the upper incisors;

1.2.2.2 *Dento-alveolar*, with more or less marked incisor protrusion, so that usually a combined form of tooth movement (bodily and tipping) will be required;

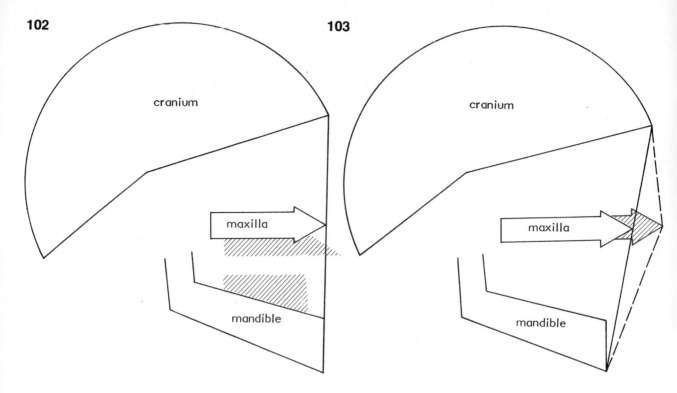

Fig. 102. Dento-alveolar Class II; diagrammatic.

Fig. 103. Anterior position of maxilla with retrognathic profile.

1.2.2.3 *A purely dental* proclination, with the upper incisors showing extreme forward inclination. Tipping the upper incisors will be all the correction required.

For the differential diagnosis of this type of malocclusion, assessment of upper incisor angulation and position (relative to the NPog line) is important. Tipping, if indicated, may be achieved with simple removable appliances, whereas bodily movement represents a more sophisticated form of treatment.

1.2.3 Neuromuscular Type

This consists in posterior displacement of the mandible due to dysfunctions. For differential diagnosis, it is difficult to distinguish this type from the orthognathic type with translocated distal closure. For differential diagnosis the SNA and SNB angles are important, and also the size and morphology of the mandible (Fig. 104).

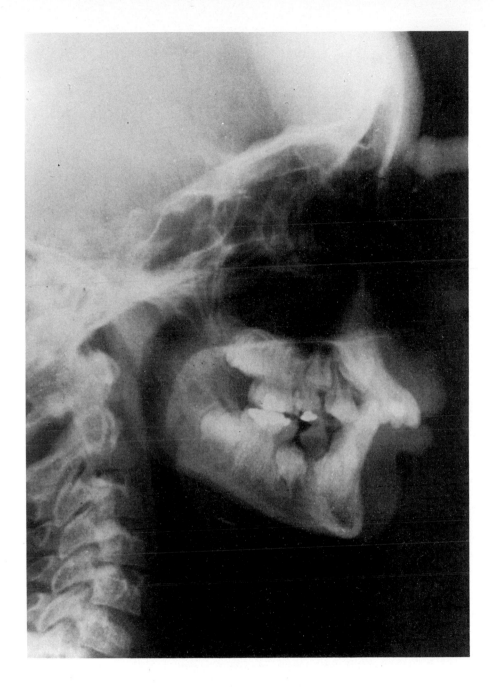

Fig. 104. Posterior displacement of mandible and protrusion of upper incisors in consequence of dysgnathia.

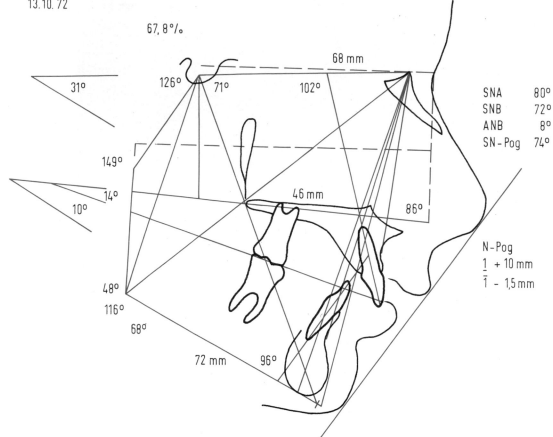

67,8%o

68 mm

31° 126° 71° 102°

SNA   80°
SNB   72°
ANB   8°
SN‑Pog 74°

149°

14°
10°

46 mm

86°

N‑Pog

$\underline{1}$ + 10 mm

$\overline{1}$ - 1,5 mm

48°
116°

68°

72 mm   96°

**Fig. 105. Posterior position of mandible, with SNB angle 72°
(mandibular base well developed) and small gonial angle (116°).**

1.2.4 Posterior Position of Maxillary and Mandibular Base

The basal structures are in a posterior position relative to the anterior cranial base, the mandible relatively more so than the maxilla. The SNA angle is small, the SNB angle even smaller. The mandible is short and retrognathic, with large saddle and articular angles, a short mandibular and small posterior cranial base (distance from sella to articulare). This is a Class II malocclusion with the 'fault in the mandible.'

1.2.4.1 The *gonial angle* may be *small*, the ascending ramus well developed. In the mixed dentition period, activator therapy may be indicated (Fig. 105).

1.2.4.2 The *gonial angle* may be *large*, the ascending ramus short and narrow. Extraction is often the treatment of choice in cases of this type, as the prognosis for forward movement of the mandible is poor (Fig. 106).

1.2.5 Combination of Groups 1.2.2 and 1.2.4

This is forward displacement of the maxilla and posterior position of the mandible (Fig. 107), so that SNA is large, SNB small. This generally calls for a combined form of treatment, e.g. headgear followed by an activator.

Cephalometric radiography provides the answers to many important questions with Class II therapy, e.g. whether movement distally or extraction is indicated,

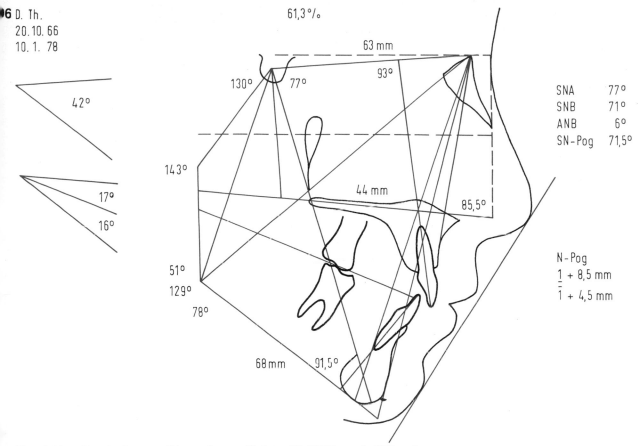

Fig. 106.   Posterior position of mandible, with SNB angle 71°, retrognathic profile, and gonial angle 129°. The lower gonial angle (Go₂) in particular is greatly enlarged (78°).

what treatment principles should be used, etc. A factor to be taken into consideration is the available forms of treatment; these are not unlimited, and some of them are in dispute. Planning must include consideration of sagittal as well as vertical relationships, as without the former it may not even be possible to produce the right bite construction for activator therapy.

 The basic principles of treatment planning for distocclusion will be discussed later.

1.3   Prognathic Skeletal Relationship

With a prognathic skeletal relationship, the maxillary and mandibular bases are anterior to the anterior cranial base. Intermaxillary relationships are usually Class III, though Class I or Class II occlusions may also be found if the mandible is large (Fig. 108).

Six types of Class III relationships may be distinguished.

1.3.1   Normal Extent of Maxillary and Mandibular Bases

The upper incisors show lingual, the lower incisors labial inclination. The cause of the anomaly can usually be localised in the dento-alveolar region. This type is often difficult to distinguish from translocated closure with marked mandibular prognathism (Fig. 109).

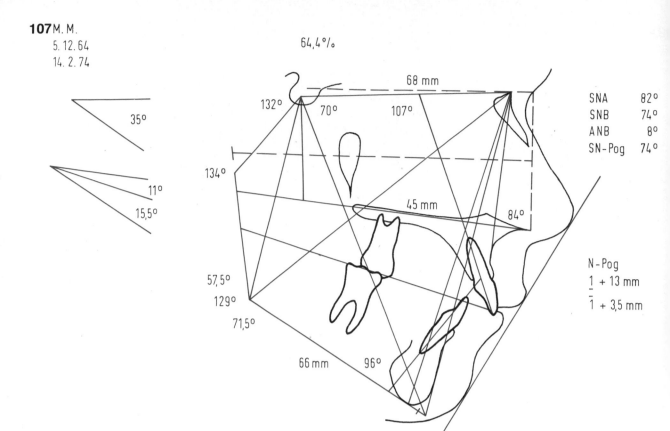

M. M.
5. 12. 64
14. 2. 74

64,4 %

35°

11°

15,5°

132° 70° 107°

134°

57,5°

129°

71,5°

68 mm

45 mm

84°

66 mm 96°

SNA   82°
SNB   74°
ANB   8°
SN-Pog 74°

N-Pog
$\underline{1}$ + 13 mm
$\overline{1}$ + 3,5 mm

Fig. 107. Combination of group 2 and 4 configuration, with forward displacement of maxilla (SNA angle 82°) and posterior position of mandible (SNB angle 74°), horizontal growth trend (64.4%). The gonial angle is 129°, as in Fig. 106, but the lower gonial angle is small (Go$_2$ = 71.5°), and the growth trend more horizontal.

108

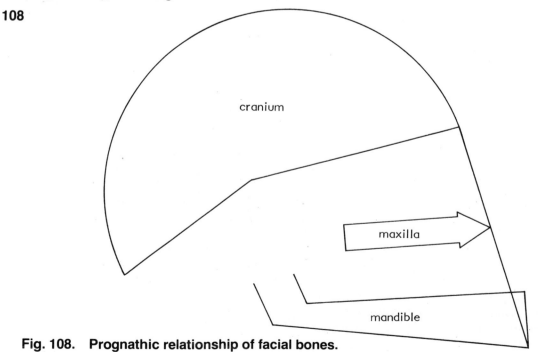

cranium

maxilla

mandible

Fig. 108. Prognathic relationship of facial bones.

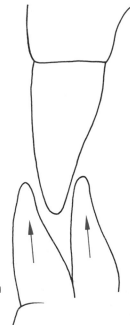

Fig. 109. **Labial tilt of the lower incisors may result in frontal cross bite.**

1.3.2 Large Mandibular Base and Ascending Ramus

The gonial angle is large, the articular angle is small. The upper incisors show labial, the lower incisors lingual inclination. Edge-to-edge or open bite are usually seen frontally, and crossbite laterally (prognathism with 'fault in the mandible'; Fig. 110).

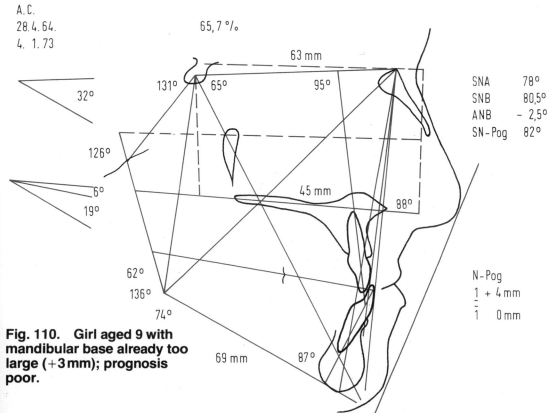

A.C.
28.4.64.
4. 1. 73

65,7 %

63 mm

131° 65° 95°

32°

126°

SNA 78°
SNB 80,5°
ANB − 2,5°
SN-Pog 82°

6°
19°

45 mm 88°

62°
136°
74°

N-Pog
$\dfrac{1}{} + 4\,mm$
$\dfrac{}{1}$ 0 mm

69 mm 87°

Fig. 110. **Girl aged 9 with mandibular base already too large (+3 mm); prognosis poor.**

1.3.3 Underdeveloped Maxilla

This presents with crowding in the upper front region, with the mandibular base prominent. Two variations of the type may be distinguished.

1.3.3.1 *Vertical growth tendency*. The ascending ramus and posterior cranial base are short, the gonial angle large, the upper gonial angle (Go_1) greater than 62° (Fig. 111a, b, see page 128).

1.3.3.2 *Horizontal growth tendency*. The ascending ramus and posterior cranial base are large, the gonial angle is small, the upper gonial angle (Go_1) 40–55° (Fig. 112a, b, see page 129).

The crowding in the maxilla complicates treatment with these two types, so that fixed appliances are usually required (mandibular prognathism with the 'fault in the maxilla').

1.3.4 Maxilla Underdeveloped, Mandible Normal

This type occurs with maldevelopment of the maxilla, e.g. in subjects with cleft palates and certain syndromes where mid-face underdevelopment is characteristic (mandibular prognathism with the 'fault in the maxilla').

1.3.5 Maxilla Normal, Mandible Overdeveloped

This group includes 'genuine' mandibular prognathism, with a poor prognosis for effective treatment (prognathism with the 'fault in the mandible'; Fig. 113).

1.3.6 Pseudo Translocated Closure

A fully developed skeletal prognathism may be partly compensated by lingual inclination of the lower and labial inclination of the upper incisors. On clinical examination, the anomaly gives the impression of being a translocated closure, but cephalometric radiography and 'mental repositioning' of incisor angulation will reveal a genuine mandibular prognathism (Fig. 144).

Even in adults, translocated closures are sometimes difficult to distinguish from true prognathism. Patient M.G., 28 years of age, has a genuine prognathism (Fig. 115), but is nevertheless able to compensate this and achieve edge-to-edge bite, though there is no contact laterally (Fig. 116).

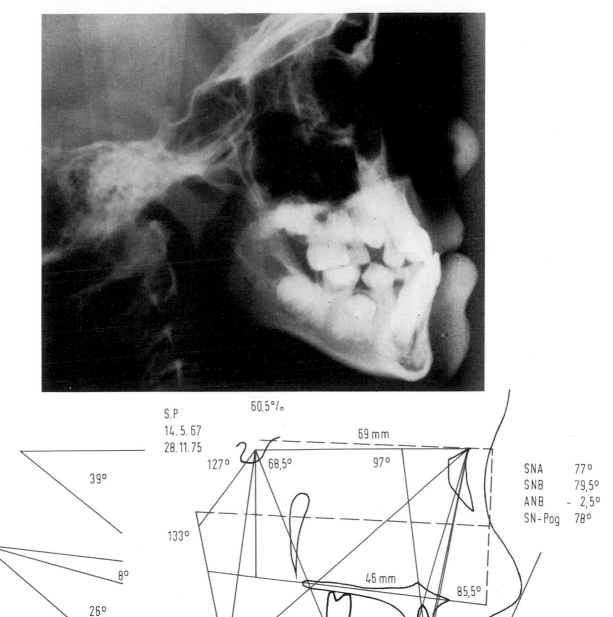

S.P.
14. 5. 67
28. 11. 75

60,5°/₀ → 60,5 %

127° 68,5° 97°

69 mm

39°

8°

26°

133°

46 mm 85,5°

60°
142°
82°

68 mm 88°

SNA 77°
SNB 79,5°
ANB − 2,5°
SN-Pog 78°

N-Pog
1 + 3 mm
1 + 6,5 mm

Fig. 111.   Prognathism, with fault in the maxilla. SNB angle normal,
SNA angle 77°, upper and lower gonial angles large. (a) Radiograph,
(b) tracing.

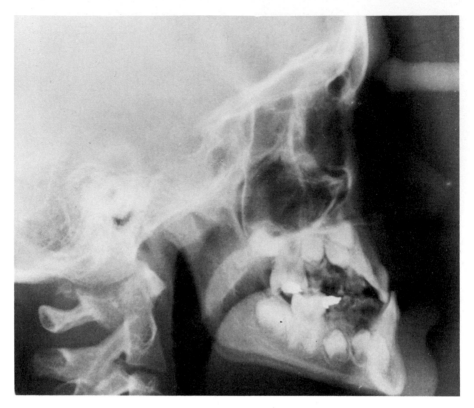

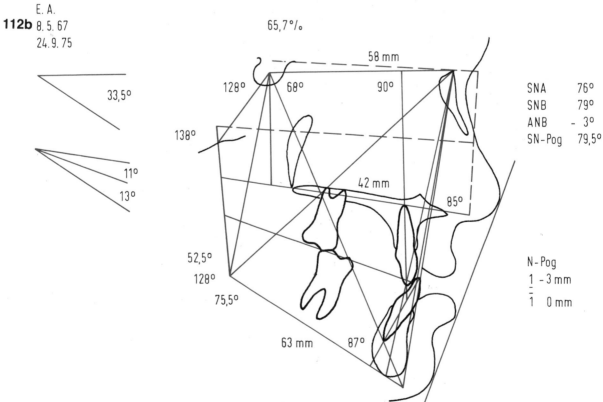

112a

E. A.
112b 8. 5. 67
24. 9. 75

65,7 %

58 mm

128° 68° 90°

138°

33,5°

11°
13°

42 mm

85°

52,5°
128°
75,5°

63 mm 87°

SNA 76°
SNB 79°
ANB − 3°
SN–Pog 79,5°

N–Pog
1 – 3 mm
1̄ 0 mm

Fig. 112.   Prognathism, with fault in the maxilla. SNA angle 76°, SNB angle 79°. Upper and lower gonial angles small. (a) Radiograph, (b) tracing.

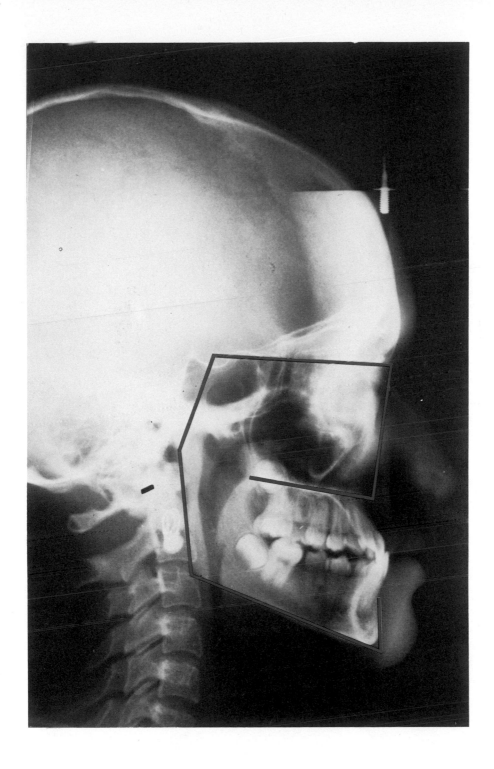

Fig. 113. Prognathism with fault in the mandible.

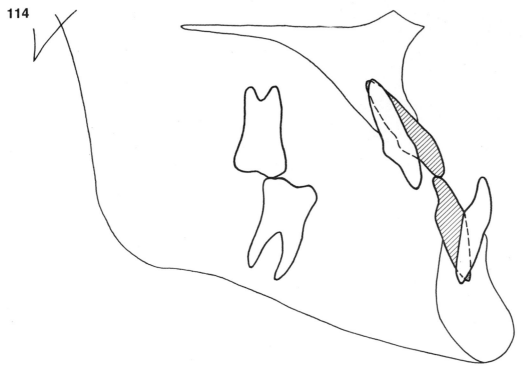

114

Fig. 114. Genuine prognathism, partly compensated by incisor angulation. The result is a pseudo-translocation.

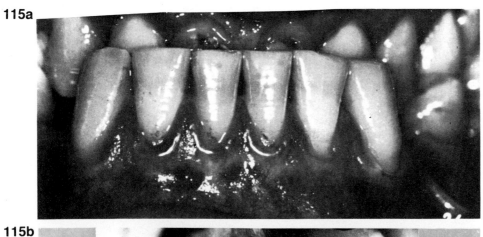

115a

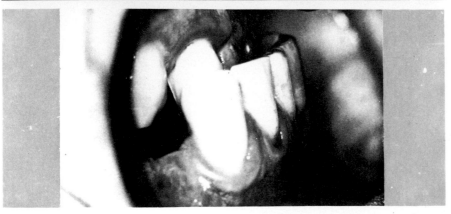

115b

Fig. 115. Genuine prognathism in a male patient aged 28. (a) Anterior view of mouth, (b) lateral view of mouth, (c) radiograph, (d) tracing, with ANB angle 10°, prognathism with the fault mainly in the mandible, and horizontal profile.

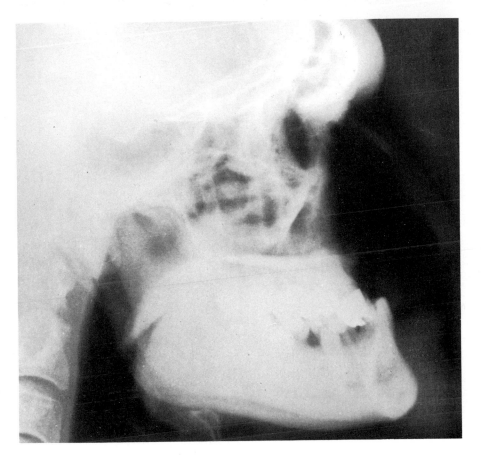

5c

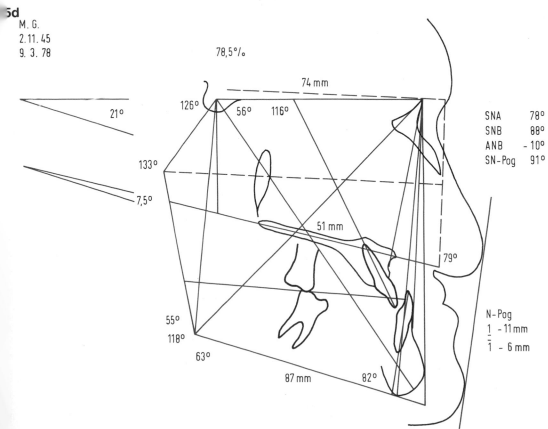

5d

M. G.
2. 11. 45
9. 3. 78

78,5%

74 mm

126°   56°   116°

21°

133°

7,5°

51 mm

79°

55°
118°

63°

87 mm   82°

SNA   78°
SNB   88°
ANB   −10°
SN-Pog 91°

N-Pog
1 − 11 mm
1̄ − 6 mm

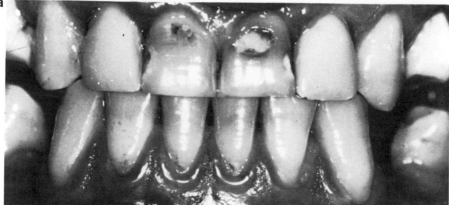

116a

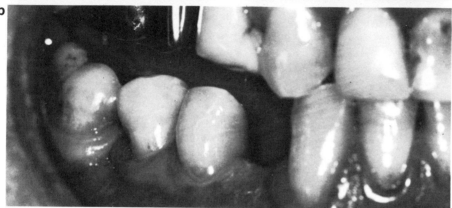

116b

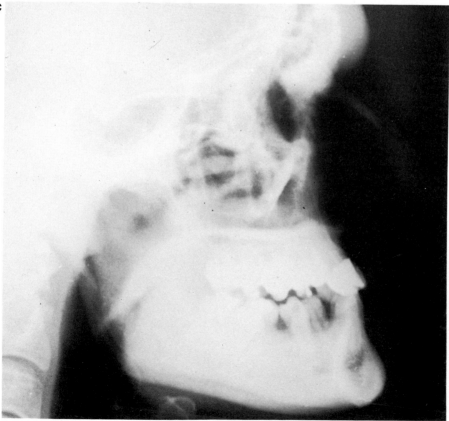

116c

Fig. 116. The same patient with maximum retraction of mandible. (a) Frontal overbite minimal, (b) open bite laterally, (c) radiograph, (d) tracing. ANB angle decreased by 6° (to 4°), SNB angle reduced to 82°. This genuine prognathism partly presents the appearance of translocation.

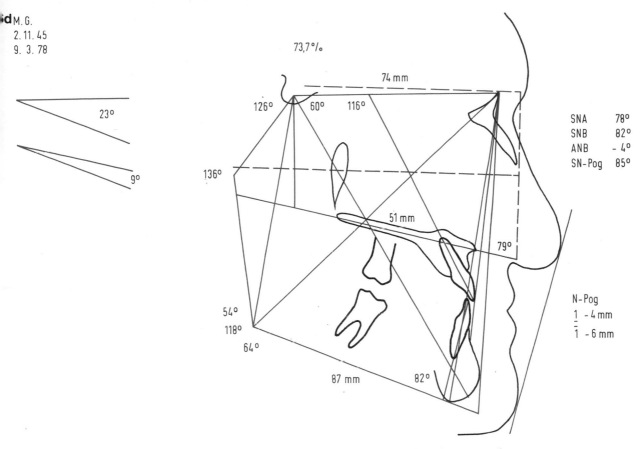

1.4 Age and Treatment-Related Changes in Cases of Prognathic Relationship

The differences between the different types of mandibular prognathism are not as highly significant at later ages than during the mixed dentition period. For example in a case of prognathism with the fault in the mandible (the body of the mandible being too long and anterior in position), a maxilla of normal size will be retarded in its further development, whilst in prognathism with the fault in the maxilla (the maxillary base being too short and in a posterior position), the mandible, having been normal in size initially, will become too long with age. This assumption has been confirmed by follow-up examination of our Class III patients.

The extent of the maxillary base and its rate of growth were small in these cases (Table 16). Some extension was achieved with treatment; the younger the patient, the more significant was the difference. The extent of the base could be changed with treatment up to the 10th year of age (i.e. with treatment initiated during the 9th year).

In the older age groups, the maxillary base did not change with treatment (Fig. 117).

The mandibular base was smaller than the average value in children with prognathism who were in their 6th and 7th years of age; after that, it was larger than the average (Fig. 118). Treatment produced no significant changes, but it is an advantage to initiate treatment at a time when the mandibular base is still relatively small in order to control the dento-alveolar growth potential. A large mandibular base was seen from the 8th year onward in our patients. The mandibular base shows a marked tendency to grow in patients with mandibular prognathism.

Dentition	Mean duration of treatment in months	Extent of mandible in mm			Ascending ramus in mm		Extent of maxilla in mm	
		Ideal	Found, before treatment*	Found, after treatment**	Found, before treatment*	Found, after treatment**	Found, before treatment*	Found, after treatment**
Primary dentition								
Fault in mandible	7	61.6±1.1	+2.0±1.0	+0.9±1.8	0 ±2.3	+2.6	+0.2±1.0	+0.5
Fault in maxilla	18	65.7±1.9	−4.2±2.4	+1.5±1.2	−2.7±1.3	+2.0	−5.0±1.0	+4.21±1.2
Together	13	64.0±1.7	−1.4±2.1	−0.9±2.0	−1.5±1.8	+2.2	−2.8±1.2	+2.8±1.4
Mixed dentition								
Fault in mandible	6.2	64.0±2.2	+4.9±2.3	+0.6±1.0	−0.4±1.5	+1.4	−0.3±1.4	+0.7
Fault in maxilla	10	67.6±2.6	−2.1±2.2	+1.0±1.0	0.0±1.6	+0.7	−3.0±2.4	+0.7
Together	9	65.7±2.1	+1.4±2.4	+0.6±1.0	−0.4±1.5	+1.4	−1.4±2.0	+0.7±2.3
Permanent dentition								
Fault in mandible	15	66.2±1.2	+6.4±3.4	∅	+6.5±3.2	+0.6	0.0±1.0	∅
Fault in maxilla	8	70.5±3.1	+0.5±3.0	∅	+4.6±3.6	∅	−2.0±2.2	∅
Together	14	68.5±3.5	+0.5±3.0	∅	+6.0±2.5	∅	−1.5±1.5	∅

* Relative to 'ideal' values.
** Relative to 'found' values prior to treatment.

Table 16. Extent of mandibular base, maxillary base, and length of ascending ramus in cases of prognathism.

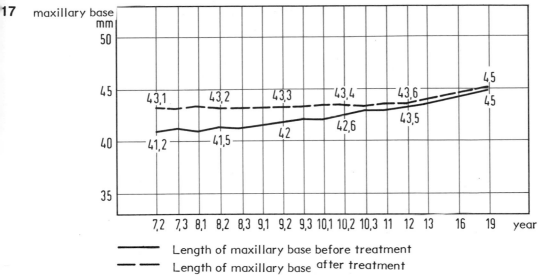

17

Length of maxillary base before treatment
Length of maxillary base after treatment

Fig. 117. **Changes in length of maxillary base with age and in the course of treatment.**

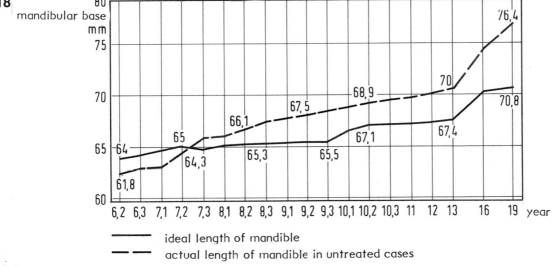

18

ideal length of mandible
actual length of mandible in untreated cases

Fig. 118. **Changes in length of mandibular base in cases of prognathism, relative to age and ideal values.**

The length of the ascending ramus was compared to the ideal values before and after treatment. Prior to treatment, it was shorter than the relevant average from the 6th to the 8th year, after which its extent increased proportionally with age (Fig. 119).

Our investigations have shown that the best possible time for initiating treatment for prognathism is the period of primary dentition, before the permanent incisors erupt. At that point it is still possible to have considerable influence on the development of the maxilla and achieve correct incisor angulation.

In the case of patient H.I., a four-year-old boy, activator therapy was initiated for prognathism. The activator had a special construction, with pads in the upper labial sulcus and a tongue guard in the mandibular portion. Normal overbite was achieved after four months of treatment (Fig. 120, 121).

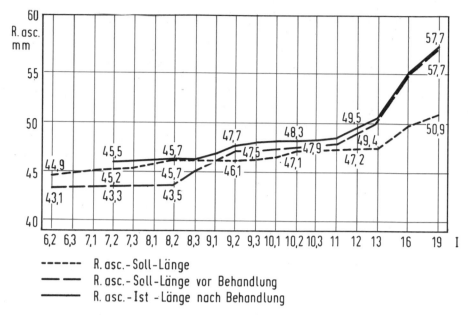

119

R.asc.–Soll–Länge

R.asc.–Soll–Länge vor Behandlung

R.asc.–Ist–Länge nach Behandlung

Fig. 119. Changes in length of ascending ramus in cases of prognathism, relative to age and during treatment compared to ideal values.

120

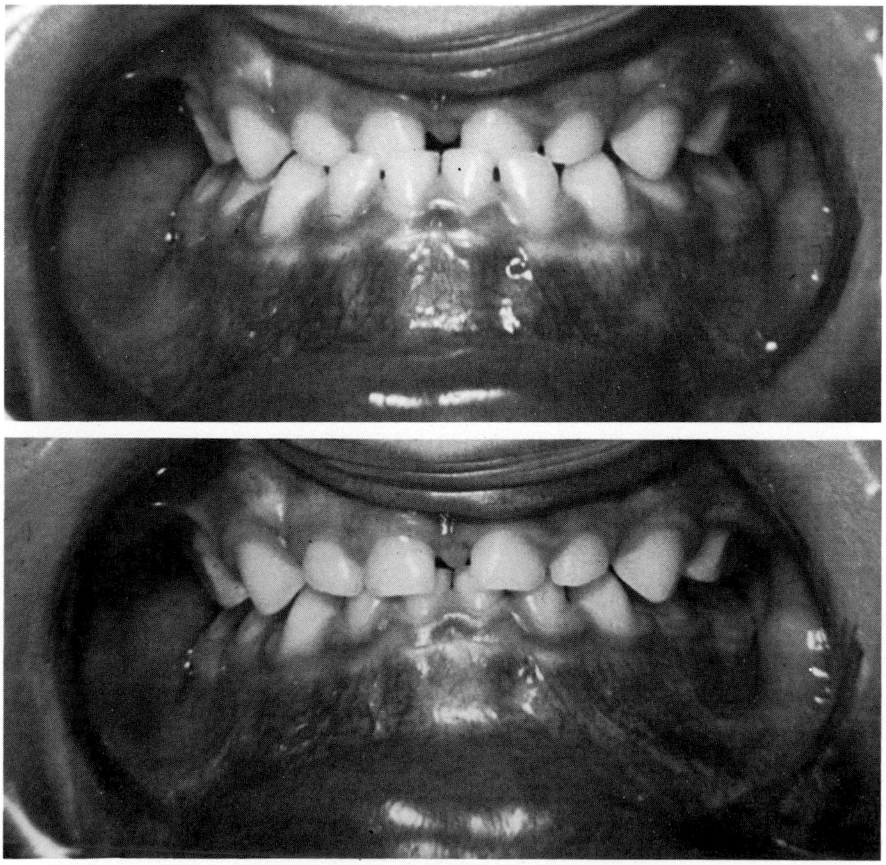

Fig. 120. Treatment of prognathism in a 4-year-old girl. Above, before treatment, below, after 8 months treatment.

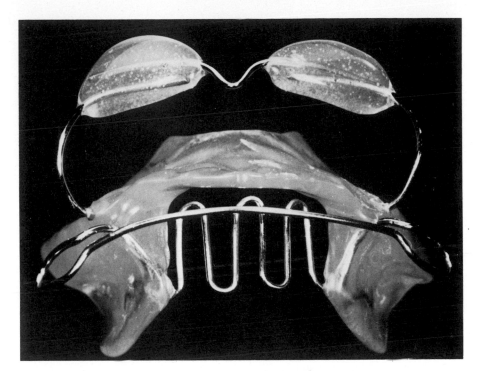

Fig. 121.   Activator for prognathism, with pads in the maxillary and tongue screen in the mandibular region.

If treatment is again required at the mixed dentition stage, the prognathic symptoms are no longer so marked as a rule.

Reversal of a frontal cross-bite had also been achieved in the case of E.K., a five-year-old girl, duration of treatment being 8 months (Fig. 122). The family then went abroad and treatment was discontinued. The patient returned at age 12, when the family had moved back to this country, with a minor degree of crowding in the upper and lower jaws (Fig. 123). Cephalometric radiography revealed no sign of Class III malocclusion (Fig. 124). The position of the mandible was prognathic, but this was compensated in the maxilla, the SNA angle being 85.5°. Early treatment had enabled the maxilla to develop to this extent.

Our investigations have however shown that certain relationships can still be influenced at the stage of early mixed dentition. Treatment of mandibular prognathism will usually still be effective from the 7th to the 9th year with no risk of creating traumatising occlusion. Even at a later age, treatment offers some prospect of success, but the later it is initiated, the greater is the risk of a relapse and therefore also the incidence of late damage.

1.5   Correlative Comparison of Sagittal Malocclusions

The differentiation of various forms of Class III malocclusions as shown above can be made only on the basis of correlative assessment of the various relationships. Seen in isolation, skeletal dimensions are not pathognomic for mandibular prognathism. A large mandible, for example, may occur in conjunction with Class II malocclusion, or a Class III facial type with normal occlusion.

Comparison of serial analyses of Class II and III shows that the differences between the two groups arise only through combination of a number of individual variations (Fig. 125a, b).

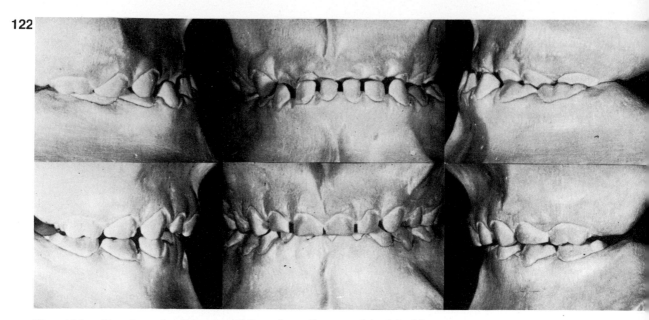

Fig. 122. Treatment of prognathism in a 5-year-old girl. Above, before treatment, below, after treatment.

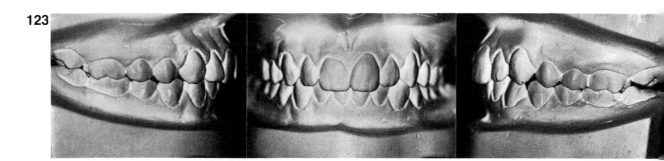

Fig. 123. Patient from Fig. 122 in her 12th year, when permanent dentition was complete.

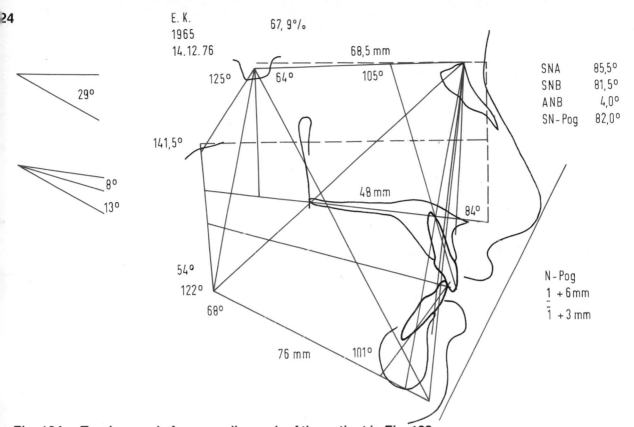

E. K.
1965
14.12.76

67, 9%

68,5 mm

125° 64° 105°

141,5°

48 mm

84°

54°
122°

68°

76 mm   101°

SNA   85,5°
SNB   81,5°
ANB   4,0°
SN-Pog 82,0°

N-Pog
$\frac{1}{\overline{1}}$ +6mm
      +3 mm

Fig. 124.   Tracing made from a radiograph of the patient in Fig. 123. Prognathic profile. Prognathism of the lower face was compensated by subsequent development of the midface.

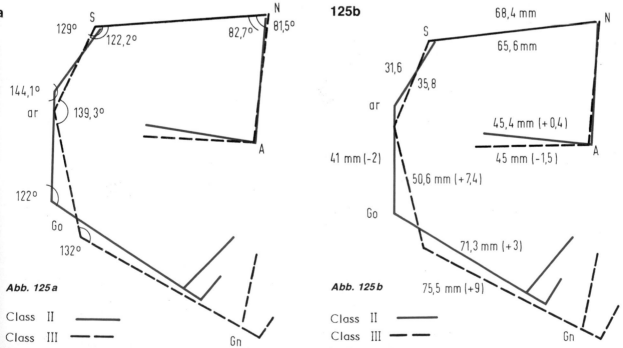

125b

a

129° S 122,2°   N 81,5°
                  82,7°

144,1°
ar   139,3°

A

122°

Go

132°

Abb. 125a

Class II ———
Class III ― ― ―
                              Gn

125b

S   68,4 mm   N
     65,6 mm

31,6
     35,8

ar

45,4 mm (+0,4)

41 mm (-2)   45 mm (-1,5)   A

50,6 mm (+7,4)

Go

71,3 mm (+3)

Abb. 125b   75,5 mm (+9)

Class II ———
Class III ― ― ―
                              Gn

Fig. 125.   Mean values for Class II and Class III skeletal relationships, shown in diagrammatic form and superimposed along the SN line. (a) Angular, (b) linear mean values.

29°

8°
13°

129

2 Assessment of Vertical Relationships in the Facial Skeleton

Assessment of facial types is mainly based on sagittal relationships (to determine orthognathic, retrognathic and prognathic conformations). To determine the facial type, assessment of sagittal relationships must be combined with that of vertical relationships. We therefore use not only the established nomenclature (orthognathic etc.), but also make the distinction regarding vertical and horizontal facial type. The reason is that the direction of mandibular growth relative to the cranial or maxillary base may differ.

2.1 Growth-Related Rotation of the Mandible

The direction of growth depends on the relative rate of growth in the condylar, sutural, and alveolar regions. If growth in the posterior face (condylar growth) is in equilibrium with growth in the anterior face (growth in the facial sutures and alveolar growth), the result is a parallel growth displacement involving no rotation. Increased growth in the anterior region (sutural alveolar) causes backward rotation (vertical growth direction), increased growth in the posterior region (condylar) causes forward rotation (horizontal growth direction) (Fig. 126).

126

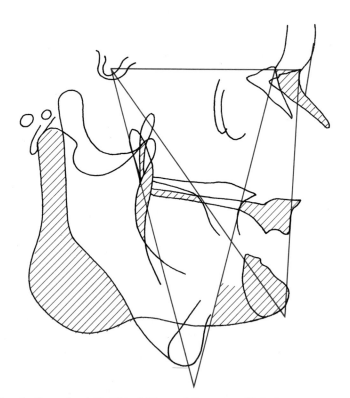

Fig. 126. **Horizontal (shaded) and vertical rotation of the mandible; diagram.**

The facial skeleton shows completely different relationships with vertical and horizontal growth types.

2.1.1 Vertical Growth Pattern

With the vertical growth type, the sum of posterior angles, the lower gonial and basal plane angles, and the angle between anterior cranial base and mandibular plane are large. Interpolation between posterior and anterior face height shows a shift favouring anterior face height. The ascending ramus is narrow and short, the mandibular base narrow, and the symphysis is thin (Fig. 127).

2.1.2 Horizontal Growth Pattern

With the horizontal growth type, the difference between posterior and anterior face height is less, so that the horizontal reference lines are more parallel. The sum of posterior angles and the basal plane angle are small, the ascending ramus is wide and long, the symphysis is wide (Fig. 128).

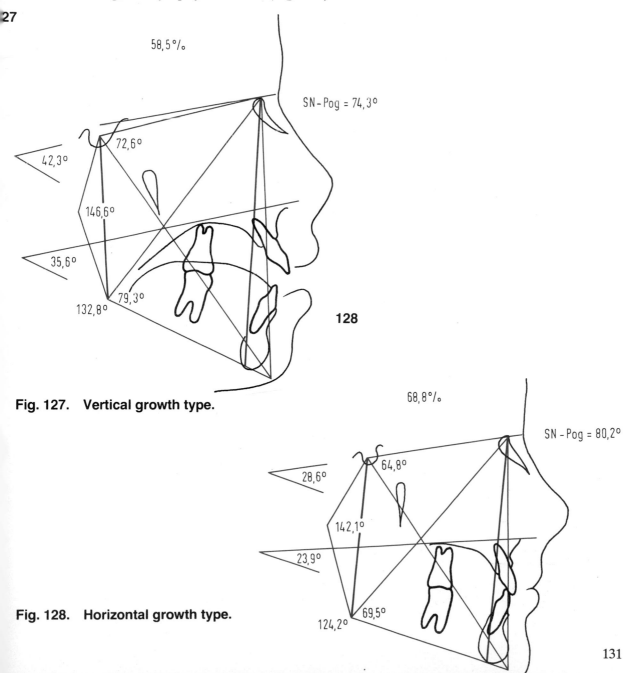

Fig. 127. Vertical growth type.

Fig. 128. Horizontal growth type.

2.1.3   Measurements in the Dento-Alveolar Region

Additional measurements taken in the dento-alveolar region permit the further analysis of vertical relationships, giving them in percentage figures (Fig. 129, Biggerstaff et al., 1977).

In the maxilla

$$\frac{\text{Perpendicular from mesial cusp of upper 6th to palatal plane} \times 100}{\text{Perpendicular from inc.sup. to palatal plane}}\%$$

The mean values are 91% for boys, and 89% for girls.

In the Mandible

$$\frac{\text{Perpendicular from mesial cusp of lower 6th to mandibular plane} \times 100}{\text{Perpendicular from inc.inf. to mandibular plane}}\%$$

The mean values are 75% at age 12 and 78% at age 16.

129

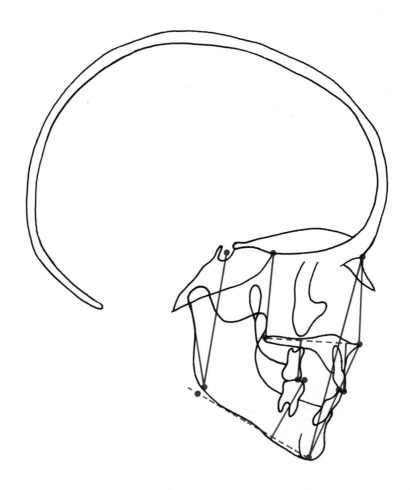

Fig. 129.   Measurements relating to incisors and 6th-year molars, for the assessment of vertical relationships in the dento-alveolar region.

2.2   Determination of the Centre of Rotation

Determination of the centre of rotation permits the finer differentiation of mandibular rotation. The centre may be located by superimposing cephalometric radiographs taken before and after treatment (Isaacson et al.).

(1) Tracings are made of the two radiographs, including the following contours: Basal plane of mandible, symphysis, posterior margin of ascending ramus, mandibular canal, lower incisors, lower sixth molar, sella, contours of forehead.

(2) On the first tracing, a reference point is found in the region of the symphysis and one in the region of the mandibular canal (Fig. 130a).

(3) The mandibular structures of the two tracings are superimposed, and the reference points transferred to the second tracing (Fig. 130b).

(4) A reference line is drawn in the region of the anterior cranial base.

(5) Now the structures of the cranial base are superimposed; the reference points no longer coincide.

(6) Corresponding reference points are joined by a line (Fig. 130c).

(7) A perpendicular is constructed on each of the lines thus produced, and the two perpendiculars are intersected. The point of intersection represents the centre of rotation (Fig. 130d).

With horizontal growth, the centre of rotation lies anterior, with vertical growth it is posterior. Its location depends also on the vector of condylar growth.

If condylar growth is upwards and forwards, the centre of rotation is low, whilst with growth directed upward and back it lies high.

With a high degree of rotation (large difference between posterior and anterior growth rate), the centre of rotation lies close to the facial structures; the smaller the difference between posterior and anterior growth rate, the farther away is the centre from these structures. In cases of translation (parallel growth), the centre lies at infinity.

2.3   The Significance of Mandibular Rotation

Mandibular rotation is a major factor in the development of malocclusion. Posterior rotation is frequently seen with retrogenia, anterior rotation with progenia.

Skeletal open bite is concomitant with posterior rotation, skeletal deep bite with forward rotation.

The variations in direction of growth giving rise to the above rotations are not only a factor in the development of malocclusions, but also play an important role in treatment planning. With forward rotation, treatment of Class III and deep bite is difficult, with backward rotation that of Class II and open bite. It is therefore important to determine the growth type before orthodontic treatment is initiated.

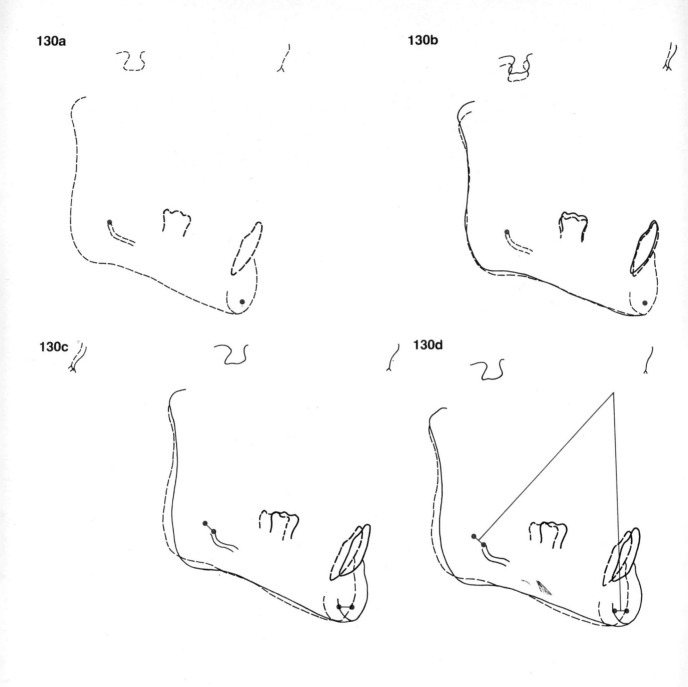

130a

130b

130c

130d

Fig. 130. Determination of centre of rotation by superposition of two radiographs, after Isaacson et al. (a) Location of reference points in the radiograph taken prior to treatment, (b) superposition of tracings along mandibular structures and transfer of reference points, (c) superposition of structures in the region of the cranial base, connecting the reference points which no longer coincide, (d) perpendiculars constructed on the lines joining the points. The point of intersection of the two perpendiculars is the centre of rotation.

2.4   Rotation of the Maxilla

Growth-related rotation may also occur in the mid-face. The nature of it may be determined along the palatal plane and expressed by the angle of inclination (Fig. 131a, b). Mid-face rotation is only partly due to growth, as it may also be affected by mechanical forces. Occlusal forces act in the cranial; gravity acts in the caudal direction; these forces may have an effect on the inclination of the maxilla. Depending on the direction of the force applied, rotation may also develop in the course of headgear therapy. It has been noted, however, that therapeutic parallel displacements of the maxilla enforced by translation are very much less liable to relapse than rotations obtained by tipping.

To assess the effect of mandibular rotation on skeletal relationships in the face, one also needs to take into account maxillary movement. Single rotations will frequently have a combined or compensatory effect, and there are a number of possible combinations.

Rotation may also be controlled, using a specially designed activator, and utilised for therapeutic purposes.

Both jaws may rotate in the same direction (horizontally or vertically) or in opposite directions (maxilla vertically, mandible horizontally, or vice versa).

2.4.1   Rotation in Opposite Directions

Horizontal rotation of the maxilla with vertical rotation of the mandible will cause the bite to open. Vertical rotation of the maxilla with horizontal rotation of the mandible will cause the bite to close.

2.4.2   Rotation in the Same Direction

The following combinations are possible with rotation in the same direction.

2.4.2.1   *Horizontal rotation of maxilla and mandible*

(a) The mandible shows greater rotation than the maxilla, resulting in closure of the bite.

(b) The maxilla shows greater rotation than the mandible, resulting in bite opening.

2.4.2.2   *Vertical rotation of maxilla and mandible*

(a) The mandible shows greater rotation than the maxilla, resulting in bite opening.

(b) The maxilla shows greater rotation than the mandible, resulting in closure of the bite.

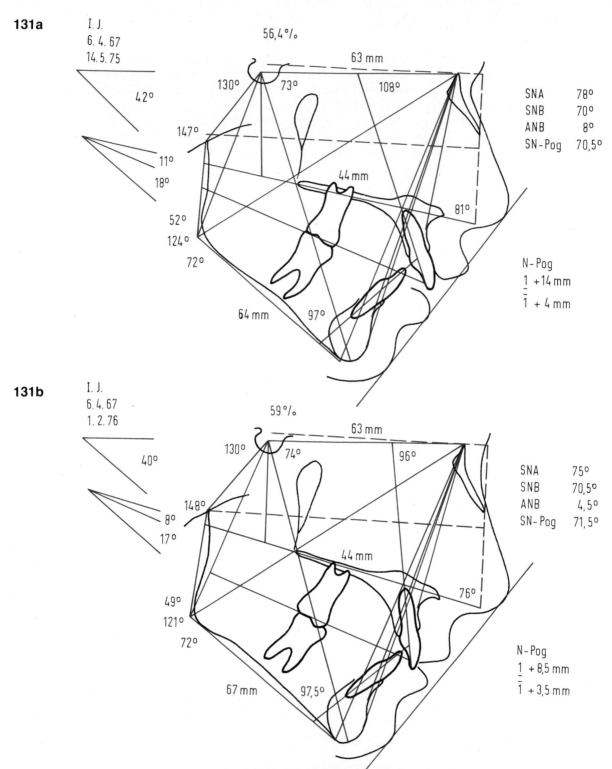

131a

I. J.
6. 4. 67
14. 5. 75

56,4%

63 mm

42°

130° 73° 108°

147°

11°

18°

44 mm

52°

124°

72°

81°

64 mm 97°

SNA 78°
SNB 70°
ANB 8°
SN-Pog 70,5°

N-Pog
$\underline{1}$ +14 mm
$\overline{1}$ + 4 mm

131b

I. J.
6. 4. 67
1. 2. 76

59%

63 mm

40°

130° 74° 96°

148°

8°

17°

44 mm

49°

121°

72°

76°

67 mm 97,5°

SNA 75°
SNB 70,5°
ANB 4,5°
SN-Pog 71,5°

N-Pog
$\underline{1}$ +8,5 mm
$\overline{1}$ +3,5 mm

Fig. 131. Change in angle of inclination indicates maxillary rotation. In vertical growth types it is frequently necessary to encourage anterior rotation of the maxilla. In the case shown here (I.J.), with vertical growth trend and ANB angle 8°, treatment achieved a 5° retro-inclination (from 81° to 76°). In this way it is possible to adapt the maxillary base to some extent to the lower dental arch. (a) Before, (b) after rotation of the maxilla.

2.5 Rotation as a Factor in Treatment Planning

The rotation of the maxillary and mandibular bases is a major factor in:

Aetiological assessment.

Determining the nature of the anomaly.

Prognostic evaluation.

Determining the possible forms of treatment and the indication.

Choosing the principles of treatment.

Assessing the stability of treatment results.

Considering the possibility and effectiveness of selective grinding of the dentition.

2.6 Horizontal Rotation of the Mandible and Deep Bite

Growth induced horizontal rotation of the mandible predestines deep bite. The mandible rotates upwards in front, increasing incisor overbite. This needs to be very much taken into account in treatment planning and post-treatment retention. With this facial type the development of tertiary crowding of the lower incisors tends to be most frequent.

Deep bite may exist also without this characteristic mandibular rotation, in which case the treatment possibilities and prognosis are totally different. The problems of treatment then have their focus in the dento-alveolar area.

Deep bite with horizontal rotation of the mandible is designated skeletal deep bite. When cephalometric radiography is used to differentiate the various forms of deep bite, one has to consider the question as to which growth processes were chiefly responsible for this development.

The development of deep bite is determined by growth changes in the following areas (Fig. 132):

(1) Temporo-mandibular joint.

(2) Maxillary base.

(3) Posterior alveolar process of maxilla.

(4) Posterior alveolar process of mandible.

(5) Vertical growth of upper anterior alveolar process.

(6) Vertical growth of lower incisors.

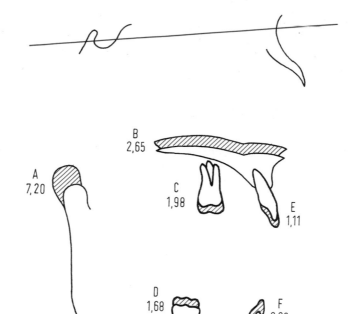

Fig. 132.   Localization and extent of growth changes involved in the development of deep bite (Schudy).

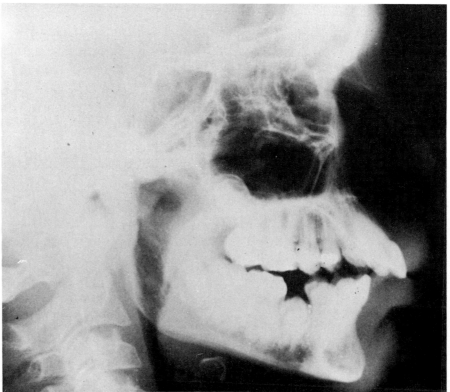

Fig. 133.   Deep bite with horizontal growth trend, short anterior face height and small interocclusal space.

Depending on the synchronisation of growth in these areas, growth-related rotation of the mandible may be forward or back. With forward rotation deep bite will become more and more serious, and it will finally be skeletal. In the teleradiograph the symptoms of deep bite are as follows (Fig. 133):

(1) Short anterior face height.

(2) Short lower face.

(3) Palatal, occlusal and mandibular planes horizontal.

(4) Gonial angle small.

(5) Basal plane angle small.

(6) Ascending ramus long and wide.

(7) Mandibular base well developed.

There is also a dento-alveolar as distinct from skeletal deep bite, with infracclusion of the molars or supracclusion of the incisors. This form may also occur in conjunction with vertical growth direction.

Correction of skeletal deep bite is possible only by movement distally or perhaps even extraction of the 2nd molars. Premolar extraction is contra-indicated with this facial type.

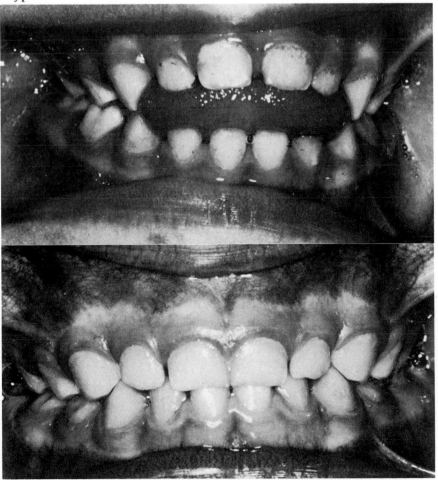

Fig. 134. **Open bite due to sucking habit. (a) Before and (b) after 4 months treatment.**

2.7   Vertical Rotation of the Mandible and Open Bite

Different forms of open bite are distinguished, and, depending on the skeletal relationships and ætiology, one may be dealing with a very simple anomaly or one that is extremely difficult to treat, with the results of treatment uncertain. Functional analysis will not give accurate differentiation of this type of anomaly. Tongue thrust is always a concomitant of open bite, irrespective of the origin of the malocclusion. The location of the open bite within the facial skeleton is a decisive factor.

Open bite due to habit is an anomaly arising through dysfunction. The anomaly may be located in the dento-alveolar region, with skeletal relationships normal. Horizontal growth is also frequently seen with anterior open bite. With this growth type, tongue pressure produces bialveolar protrusion with spacing. During the stage of mixed dentition, causal therapy may be effected by inhibition, i.e. elimination of the dysfunction (e.g. with a tongue crib).

In a five-year-old girl with open bite and a persistent sucking habit, the open bite was corrected within 4 months by eliminating the dysfunction. The direction of growth being average, further development is expected to be normal (Fig. 134a, b).

R.S., a seven-year-old girl, presented with open bite, tongue and lip dysfunction, and vertical growth type (Fig. 135a, b).

135a

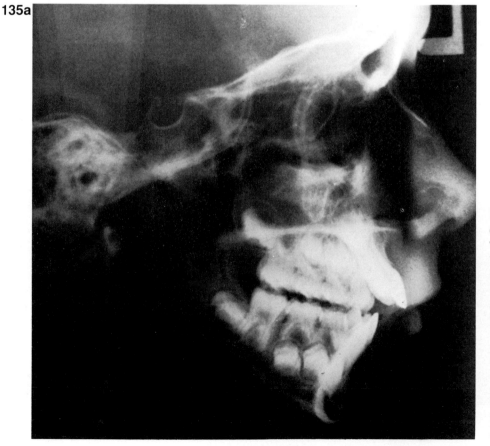

Fig. 135.   Open bite due to sucking habit with vertical growth trend in patient R.S. (a) Radiograph, (b) tracing. The ANB angle was 5°, the lower gonial angle 77.5°, the relation of posterior to anterior face height 55.5%. The first stage of treatment was designed to eliminate the adverse pressures by inhibition (vestibular appliance).

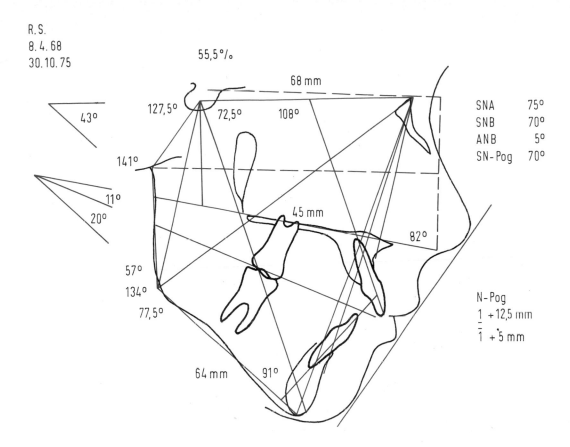

R.S.
8.4.68
30.10.75

55,5%

68 mm

43°

127,5°   72,5°   108°

141°

11°
20°

45 mm

82°

57°
134°

77,5°

64 mm   91°

SNA   75°
SNB   70°
ANB   5°
SN-Pog 70°

N-Pog
1 +12,5 mm
1 + 5 mm

Despite the vertical growth pattern, treatment was initiated with a vestibular screen, to eliminate the dysfunction. After one year of treatment, maxillary relationships were normal, the open bite corrected, and the ANB angle reduced from 5° to 2°. A vestibular screen will have no direct effect on vertical growth. Correction or elimination of the dysfunction should however lead to improvement in the further development of the facial skeleton (Fig. 136a, b).

2.7.1 Skeletal Open Bite

Treatment is much more difficult with skeletal open bite where the cause is developmental and located in the skeletal region. In this anomaly, the sum of posterior angles – particularly the lower gonial angle – is large, also the basal plane angle. A retrognathic relationship has developed; anterior face height is long, posterior short, the ascending ramus is short. A dysfunction can cause a very upright position of the lower incisors.

A girl of 18 presented with skeletal open bite and maxillary as well as mandibular crowding (Fig. 137a–d). At this age, dento-alveolar compensation of the skeletal discrepancy or surgery are the only possibilities. The direction of growth was extremely vertical, 56.3%, and the lower gonial angle 85°. The upper incisors were far ahead (+ 17 mm) of the NPog line. The four first premolars were extracted, the upper and lower dental arches aligned, and the open bite corrected with the aid of intermaxillary elastics. This achieved purely dento-alveolar correction and compensation. The skeletal relationships did not change (Fig. 138a–c).

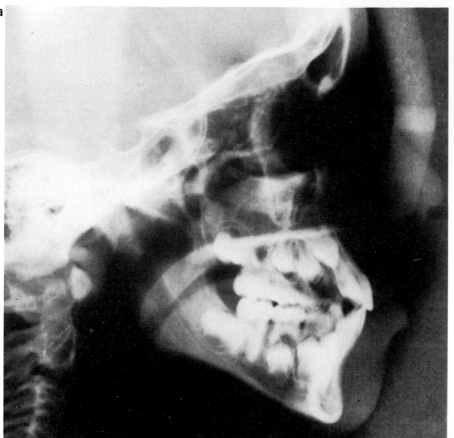

136a

Fig. 136. Patient R.S. after elimination of adverse pressures. (a) Radiograph, (b) tracing. The ANB angle has become normal, with 2°, the relation of posterior to anterior face height was 57.5%, the gonial angle enlarged. Vertical growth trends persisted after elimination of the dyskinesia. Further development needs to be monitored, so that the second stage of treatment may be timed correctly.

136b R.S.

8.4.68
28.1.77

57,5°/o

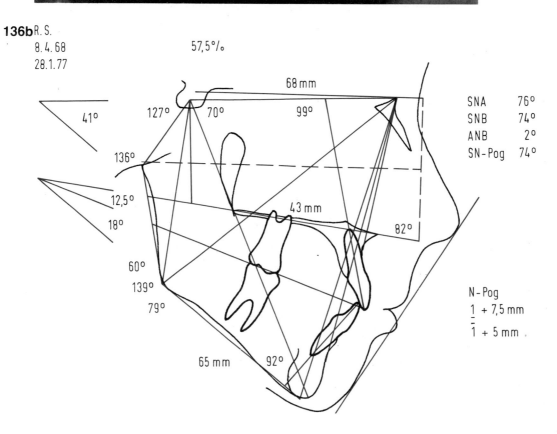

68 mm

41°   127°   70°   99°

136°

12,5°

18°   43 mm

60°

139°   82°

79°

65 mm   92°

SNA	76°
SNB	74°
ANB	2°
SN-Pog	74°

N-Pog

$\underline{1}$ + 7,5 mm

$\overline{1}$ + 5 mm

a

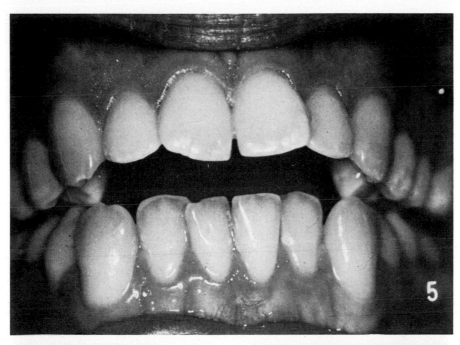

b

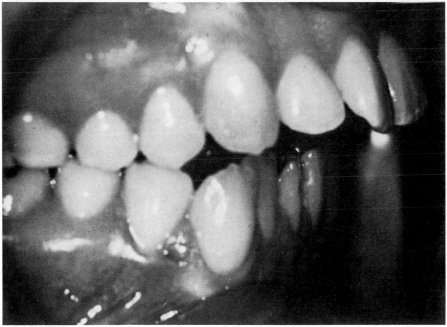

Fig. 137. With skeletal open bite in permanent dentition only active mechanical therapy is possible, with the possibility of achieving dento-alveolar compensation of the skeletal deviation. Open bite (a) in anterior view, (b) in lateral view showing marked overjet. (c) Radiograph and (d) tracing. The radiograph (c) and tracing (d) show the ANB differential to be 6.5°, relation of posterior to anterior face height 56.3%, extremely large lower gonial angle (85°).

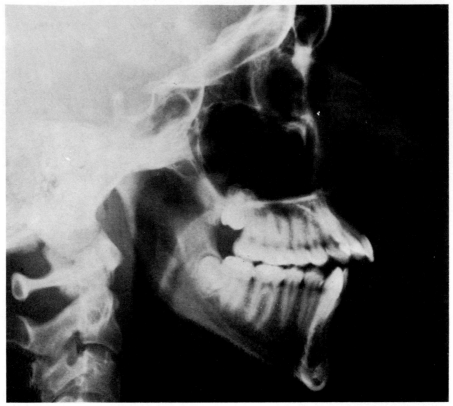

56,3%

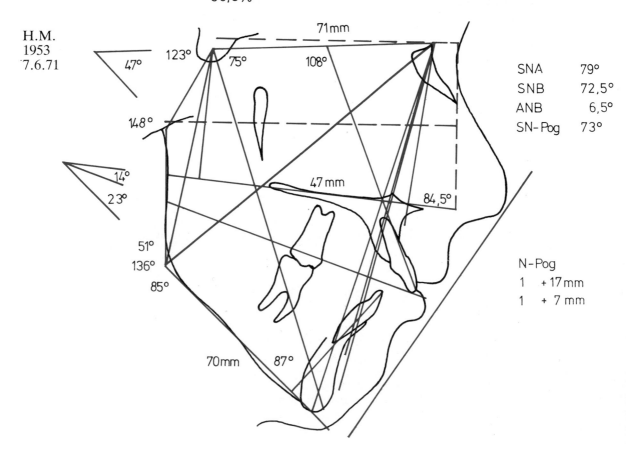

H.M.
1953
7.6.71

SNA	79°
SNB	72,5°
ANB	6,5°
SN-Pog	73°

N-Pog

1 + 17 mm

1 + 7 mm

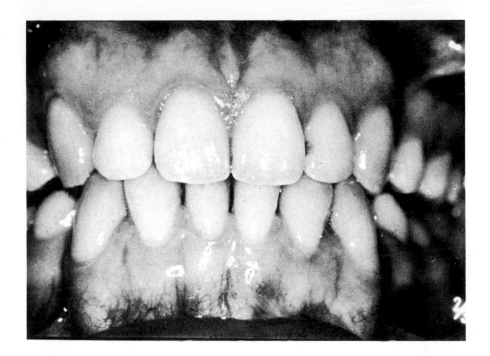

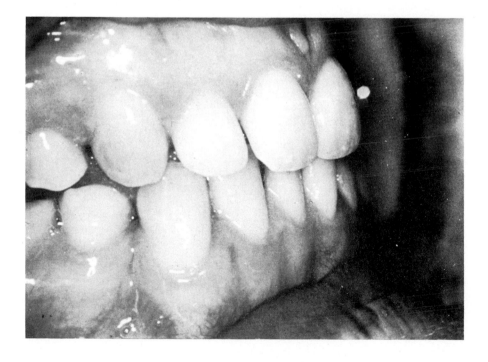

Figure. 138.   Patient H.M. after dento-alveolar compensation of the skeletal discrepancy. (a) Anterior view, (b) lateral view. The tracing (c) shows a change in the skeletal structures; following extraction of the four first premolars, the upper and lower dental arches were re-shaped, with a fixed appliance, and dento-alveolar compensation of the open bite was achieved.

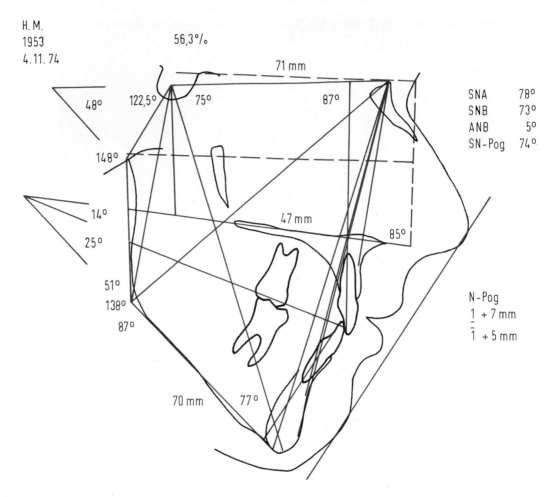

H. M.
1953
4.11.74

56,3°/₀

71 mm

48°   122,5°   75°   87°

148°

14°

25°

51°
138°
87°

70 mm   77°

47 mm

85°

SNA   78°
SNB   73°
ANB   5°
SN-Pog   74°

N-Pog
1 + 7 mm
1 + 5 mm

2.7.2   Open Bite Syndrome

A vertical growth tendency may, due to summation of a number of factors, lead to severe skeletal open bite showing progressive tendencies. Sucking habits and abnormal nasal breathing may cause further serious deterioration in the condition, so that one may speak of an open bite syndrome which may be defined as follows:

(a) Vertical growth direction; the expression of skeletal open bite.

(b) Convexity of palatal plane; the consequence of a strong sucking habit persisting for years.

(c) Antegonial notching; the expression of abnormal nasal breathing with lack of space in the epipharynx (Fig. 139).

Treatment possibilities are severely limited with a skeletal open bite. Causal therapy is not possible. The only possibility still open is dento-alveolar compensation of the skeletal deviation. Premolar extractions have a positive effect by closing the bite, providing we can effect mesial movement of the teeth behind the extraction space. In extreme cases surgery is indicated.

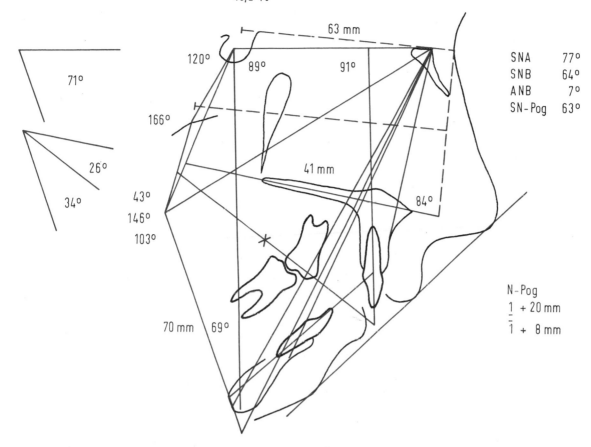

43,2 %

71°

120°   89°   91°

63 mm

166°

26°

41 mm

43°
146°
103°

84°

34°

70 mm   69°

SNA   77°
SNB   64°
ANB   7°
SN–Pog   63°

N–Pog
$\underline{1}$ + 20 mm
$\overline{1}$ + 8 mm

Fig. 139. Skeletal open bite with vertical growth type. The upper gonial angle is 146°, the lower gonial angle 103°; combination of a number of factors may produce an extreme case of open bite, so that one may speak of an Open Bite Syndrome.

3   Classification of Facial Types

The classification of facial patterns deviating from the norm comprises four basic types (modified after Sassouni).

(1) Retrognathic type (Class II).

(2) Prognathic type (Class III).

(3) Horizontal type (deep bite).

(4) Vertical type (open bite).

Combination of these types will give four more (Fig. 140):

(1) Retrognathic type with horizontal growth tendency.

(2) Retrognathic type with vertical growth tendency.

(3) Prognathic type with horizontal growth tendency.

(4) Prognathic type with vertical growth tendency.

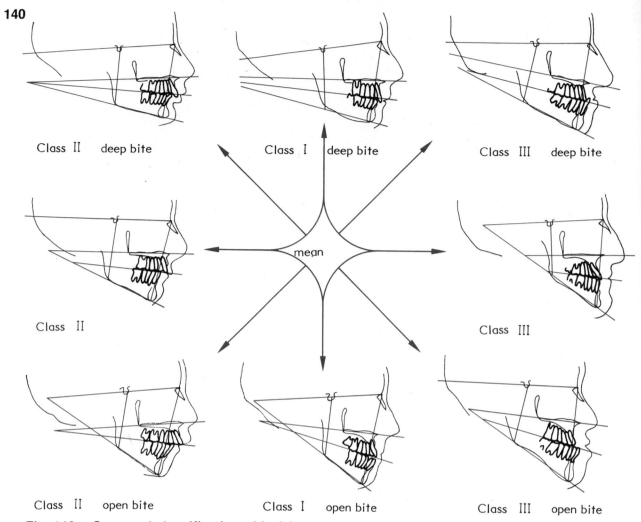

Class II   deep bite   Class I   deep bite   Class III   deep bite

Class II   mean   Class III

Class II   open bite   Class I   open bite   Class III   open bite

Fig. 140.   Sassouni classification of facial types.

Determining the classification of an anomaly under examination is an important element in both treatment planning and diagnostic assessment.

(1) With a Class II anomaly with horizontal growth pattern, the prognosis is good for correcting the Class II relationship but not for opening the bite.

(2) With a Class II anomaly with vertical growth tendency, the prognosis is good for correcting deep overbite but not the Class II relationship.

(3) With a Class III anomaly with horizontal growth pattern, the prognosis is good for correcting the Class III relationship but not the deep bite (if this should need correction).

(4) With a Class III anomaly with vertical growth tendency, the prospects for effective treatment are altogether poor.

Cephalometric Radiography and Growth

In orthodontics particular importance attaches to the significance and assessment of growth and also of function, two concepts that frequently need to be considered together. In the context of cephalometric radiography, brief mention shall at least be made of the problems arising through growth. The method is frequently used for the assessment of growth, though it cannot provide all the information required in treatment planning. The most important questions to be considered in this context are the following:

1 How Much Further Growth May be Expected

Quantitative assessment of growth is an important element in treatment planning. With younger children more growth is to be expected. The estimated growth rate will be even greater if the biological age of the child is less than its chronological age. For example, a greater rate of growth would be expected in a ten-year-old child with a biological age of nine than in a ten-year-old whose biological age is also ten. The changes that treatment can effect in skeletal relationships will largely depend on this question.

The biological age may be determined by a number of methods. The most widely used method is evaluation of the radiograph of a hand. Ossification of the carpal bones – as distinct from the long bones of the extremities – occurs during the first years of life. Up to about ten years of age, the biological age can be determined by using the carpal index. We use the scheme given by Greulich and Pyle to evaluate the radiograph of the hand. After approximately the tenth year of life, epiphyseal lines are still discernible in the metacarpal bones, and may be seen to be gradually disappearing until growth is complete. Björk distinguishes seven growth stages from the tenth year onward in boys, and the ninth year in girls (Table 17).

2 Timetable for Growth

The individual developmental stages not only permit quantitative assessment of growth, but also provide information on another point that plays a major role in treatment planning: the timing of growth rates. It is possible to estimate when growth spurts will occur prior to puberty.

3 Localisation of Growth Rates

Increase in size shows certain correlations to growth rate in the different regions of the facial skeleton. During very active growth, a noticeable increase may be noted particularly in the following linear dimensions: N-Me, S-Gn, Ar-Gn.

The prospective rate of growth in a particular region of the facial skeleton may be estimated with the aid of Table 18. This gives the mean annual growth rates.

Stage		Object	Growth	Phase
1.	PP_2	Prox. phalanx of index finger	Width of epiphysis = width of diaphysis	Prior to max. long. growth, rate of growth slow
2.	MP_3	Middle phalanx of middle finger	Width of epiphysis = width of diaphysis	Max. long. growth imminent
3.	S	Ulnar sesamoid on metacarpophalangeal joint of thumb	Signs of ossification	As stage 2
4.	$MP_{3\ cap}$	Middle phalanx of middle finger	Encapsulation of diaphysis	Max. long. growth (betw. S and MP_3carp)
5.	DP_{3u}	Distal phalanx of middle finger	Epiphysis united	Max. long. growth over
6.	PP_{3u}	Proximal phalanx of middle finger	As stage 5	As stage 5
7.	MP_{3u}	Middle phalanx of middle finger	As stage 5	Past max. growth
8.	Rc	Distal epiphysis of radius and ulna	United	Growth complete

Table 17. Table for assessment of hand X-ray (modification of Bjork's method).

Age	S–N		S–Gn		S–Go		Ar–Gn		N–ME		Maxillary base		Mandibular base	
	M	F	M	F	M	F	M	F	M	F	M	F	M	F
8	75.2	72.3	115.8	112	70	66.4	103.4	100.7	113.6	109.5	97.8	46.8	70.5	69.8
9	0.7	0.3	2.6	2.2	1.9	2.1	2.4	1.6	2.3	2.6	0.6	0.0	1.8	1.1
10	0.9	1.3	2.9	3.4	1.7	1.7	2.3	2.8	2.8	3.0	0.8	1.6	2.0	2.5
11	1.4	0.4	2.9	1.9	1.9	0.9	2.6	2.0	2.8	1.1	1.5	1.0	2.2	1.7
12	0.1	0.6	2.7	2.6	2.6	2.6	2.3	2.6	1.8	2.1	0.8	0.3	1.3	0.8
13	1.2	0.6	3.6	2.3	2.7	2.1	2.8	1.7	3.3	2.4	0.8	1.0	2.0	1.9
14	1.0	0.5	3.2	2.2	2.3	1.8	3.0	1.9	3.7	1.6	0.6	1.1	2.5	1.9
Mean	0.88	0.61	2.98	2.43	2.15	1.7	2.56	2.1	2.78	2.1	0.8	0.8	1.9	1.5

Table 18. Annual growth gain in principal linear dimensions.

4 Direction of Growth

Another important aspect is assessment of the growth direction. Cephalometric radiography may be used to distinguish horizontal and vertical growth patterns. In extreme cases, the change in growth direction during further development is of no significance. If treatment is initiated at the stage of mixed dentition a change in growth direction cannot be excluded, except of course in extreme cases. For the purpose of prediction, we combine the results of cephalometric analysis with an assessment of mandibular morphology. A broad mandibular base and ascending ramus together with a very marked, thick symphysis suggest a change in direction toward horizontal growth, as distinct from a narrow mandible and thin symphysis which are typical for vertical growth.

5 Prediction of Growth

Some investigators have specifically considered the question of forecasting individual growth patterns. It should be possible to give an accurate forecast of growth changes on the bases of radiological evaluation of craniofacial structures (Broadbent, Brodie). The conclusions arrived at were of minor significance for the individual case.

Björk has made a differentiated analysis of growth in various skeletal regions, including the extent of individual variability. The applied prediction of growth is generally based on his work, though it is also clear that individual predictions have to be regarded with considerable caution.

5.1 Methods of Predicting Growth

A number of methods are available for a more or less detailed prediction of growth changes; these cannot go into details concerning certain aspects, such as:

(a) Age-related individual peculiarities.

(b) Growth changes in untreated cases, compared with those in treated cases, taking into account treatment mechanism and the age of the patient at the beginning of treatment.

(c) Growth changes occurring after conclusion of treatment.

Growth is not a question of simple increase in size, but a highly complex process. During orthodontic treatment, complicated changes will occur even in a region where growth is relatively quiescent, e.g. in the cranial base, examples being appositional growth at basion, remodelling in the sella and at nasion, and sutural growth in the spheno-occipital synchrondrosis.

5.1.1 Johnston Method

L.E. Johnston has produced a diagram (Fig. 141) on the assumption of regular annual changes and an average direction of growth. He states that accurate prediction can be made in 65% of cases.

Johnston developed a simplified method of generating a long-term forecast by use of a printed 'forecast grid'. Each point was advanced one grid unit per year, using a standard S-N orientation registered at S.

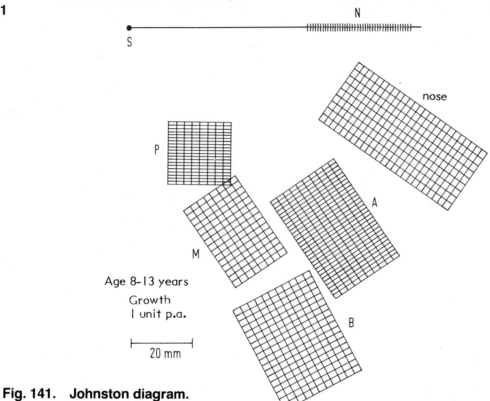

Fig. 141. Johnston diagram.

5.1.2 Growth in SN Line

A number of methods are based on the average increase in the SN line, using this for differentiated prediction of vertical and sagittal growth changes. The reliability of this method is said to be 70%. The Holdaway method belonging to this group will be described in a later chapter.

5.1.3 Ricketts' Short-Term Prediction

This makes distinction between vertical and horizontal growth. The method is said to be 80% reliable.

5.1.4 Ricketts' Computer Analysis

This considers (Fig. 142):

(a) Individual growth curves for the separate regions of the facial skeleton.

(b) Unusual growth patterns (5% of cases).

The technique used with this commercialised method has been fully documented. The basic materials are cephalometric data relating to structural synthesis stored in the computer, with a structural analysis done in the individual case. Individual assessment is again based on statistical mean values.

This computer diagnosis requires the patient to be a certain age and is also limited to specific treatment techniques. Otherwise it is difficult to explain the claim made in relation to it that, with treatment duration of two years, 70–80% of changes were due to treatment and only 20–30% to growth.

The computer can only be an aid in selecting and evaluating information within the context of treatment planning; it cannot be used to determine the actual treatment. The final decision will lie with the orthodontist who uses the computer as a source of information and as a control.

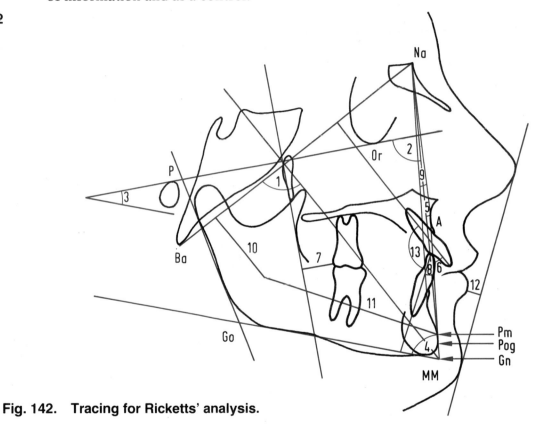

Fig. 142. Tracing for Ricketts' analysis.

5.2 Sources of Error in Growth Prediction

Growth prediction is frequently compared to the weather forecast. The prediction can be based on certain data, but so many unknown factors are involved that we can merely discern a certain trend, and not make an accurate prediction. The principal sources of error are the following:

5.2.1 Variable Growth Rate in Regional Growth Centres

Between the 8th and 14th year, for instance, the mean annual rate of increase in the maxillary base is approx. 0.8 mm, compared to 1.9 mm for the mandibular base. The growth ratio of S-N to mandibular base is 1:1.35 to 1.65, that of S-Ar to Ar-Go, 1:1.3.

5.2.2 Growth Pattern Not Fully Taken into Account

Individuals are assessed only in relation to a population mean. Many methods do not even include consideration of the growth pattern. Our own investigations have shown that growth rates will vary quite considerably for different growth types. By determining vertical increase at gonion and horizontal increase at gnathion (Fig. 143), we were able to establish the following relationship of vertical to horizontal growth: With average growth types, an increase of 1 mm vertically corresponds to one of 0.8 mm in the horizontal plane. With the vertical growth type this ratio is 1 mm : 0.3 mm, compared to 1 mm : 1.7 mm in horizontal growth types. Generally speaking, horizontal growth changes are more easily predictable than vertical changes.

143

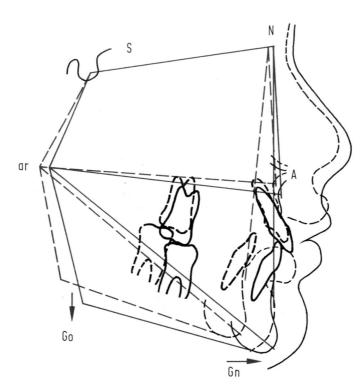

Fig. 143. Measurements to determine growth gain in the vertical direction at gonion and horizontal direction at gnathion.

5.2.3 Relationship of Form and Function

The interrelationship of form and function is not taken into consideration. A marked increase in the length of the mandible, for example, will not automatically compensate for Class II malocclusion if development is subject to interference through dysfunction.

Patient I. Ch. showed a marked increase in mandibular base. Due to persistent dysfunction, however, the condition of the malocclusion was aggravated (Fig. 144a, b).

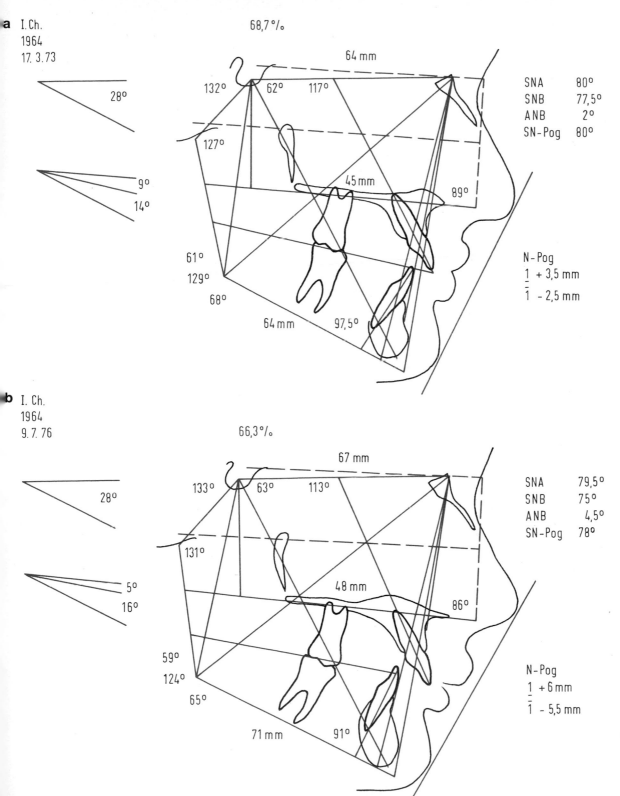

a
I.Ch.
1964
17. 3. 73

68,7 %

64 mm

132°   62°   117°

127°

45 mm

89°

61°
129°

68°

64 mm   97,5°

28°

9°
14°

SNA	80°
SNB	77,5°
ANB	2°
SN-Pog	80°

N-Pog

$\underline{1}$ + 3,5 mm

$\overline{1}$ − 2,5 mm

b
I. Ch.
1964
9. 7. 76

66,3 %

67 mm

133°   63°   113°

131°

48 mm

86°

59°
124°

65°

71 mm   91°

28°

5°
16°

SNA	79,5°
SNB	75°
ANB	4,5°
SN-Pog	78°

N-Pog

$\underline{1}$ + 6 mm

$\overline{1}$ − 5,5 mm

Fig. 144. Patient I.Ch. presented with Class II dysgnathia with horizontal growth type, and tongue and lip dysfunction. No orthodontic treatment was given (a). Despite a considerable growth gain in the mandibular base area, intermaxillary relationships became worse, due to persisting dysfunction (b).

155

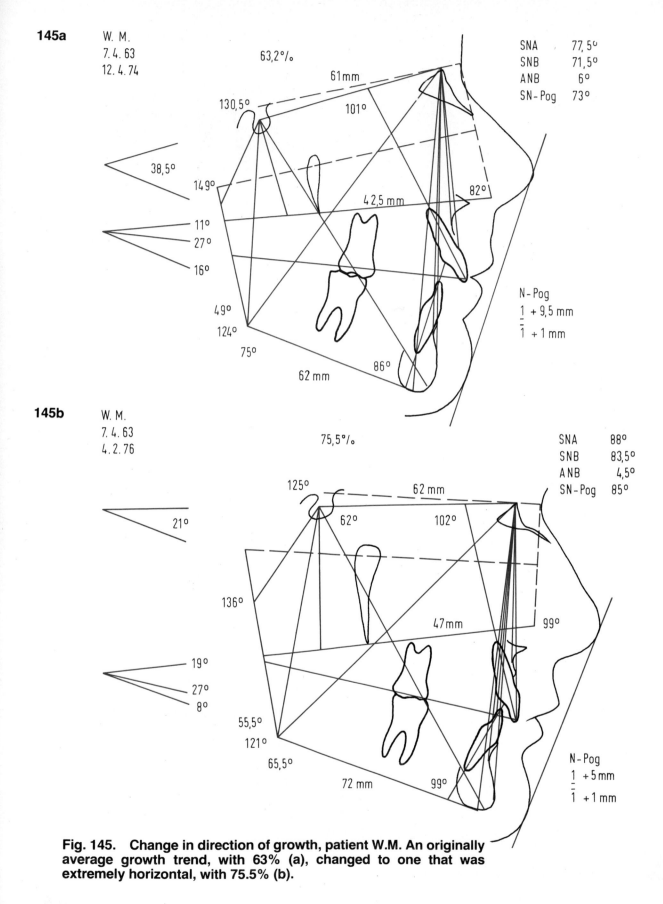

145a

W. M.
7. 4. 63
12. 4. 74

63,2%

61mm

130,5°

101°

38,5°

149°

42,5 mm

82°

11°
27°
16°

49°
124°

75°

86°

62 mm

SNA 77,5°
SNB 71,5°
ANB 6°
SN–Pog 73°

N–Pog
$\frac{1}{1}$ + 9,5 mm
$\frac{1}{1}$ + 1 mm

145b

W. M.
7. 4. 63
4. 2. 76

75,5%

125°

62 mm

21°

62°

102°

136°

47mm

99°

19°
27°
8°

55,5°
121°
65,5°

72 mm

99°

SNA 88°
SNB 83,5°
ANB 4,5°
SN–Pog 85°

N–Pog
$\frac{1}{1}$ + 5 mm
$\frac{1}{1}$ + 1 mm

Fig. 145. Change in direction of growth, patient W.M. An originally average growth trend, with 63% (a), changed to one that was extremely horizontal, with 75.5% (b).

5.2.4 Age-Related Factors

These are not usually given sufficient attention, nor the fact that before the ninth year, when the direction of growth is not yet stabilised, a change in peristasis (functional environment) will frequently cause a change in growth direction.

W.M., a girl aged 11, showed average direction of growth with open bite and Class II malocclusion (Fig. 145a, b). No orthodontic treatment was given, but two years later, when the patient returned to have the need for orthodontic treatment reassessed, the situation was totally different. The mandible had moved forward, and the rate of growth was 10 mm, with forward rotation, so that the open bite had disappeared. The direction of growth had become horizontal in the extreme. The skeletal relationship, originally retrognathic, had become prognathic. Ante-inclination (y-angle) had reduced by 16° (ante-inclination may be misinterpreted as protrusion; it is merely a pseudo-protrusion). She had a history of sucking habit, but this had stopped during the period of observation. The changes were however predominantly due to the growth spurts of puberty, and changes in the functional environment.

6 Growth Following Conclusion of Treatment

Growth prediction also serves to assess growth changes which occur after treatment has been completed. A radiograph of the hand will help to give a quantitative assessment of such changes. Cephalometric radiography enables us to estimate the consequences or effects of post-therapeutic growth phases, a significant factor for stability of results and length of retention period. The post-therapeutic changes to be expected are shown in Table 19 (the mean values given are intended as a guide only; they are not standards).

anterior growth		
point A	1.36 mm	
pogonion	3.62 mm	
condylar growth		
vertical	5.4 mm	
horizontal	1.0 mm	
gonial angle		
caudal	4.34 mm	
anterior	0.41 mm	
occlusal		Anterior growth of mandible.
$\frac{6}{6}$	1.25 mm	Decrease in:
	0.99 mm	SN–MP, ANB, B, Go angles
mesial tilt		$\underline{1}$–tilt
$\underline{6}$	7.2°	$\overline{1}$–position depending on vertical growth changes (unfavourable angulation + direction of growth = tertiary crowding).

Table 19. Mean post-therapeutic growth gains.

6.1 Fine Adjustment of Occlusion After Treatment

Post-therapeutic growth changes may affect intercuspidation and play a role in fine adjustment of the occlusion.

6.1.1 Anterior Growth of the Mandible

This occurs during the final growth phase. Its mean value in the pogonion region is 3.6 mm. The SN-Pog angle increases by 1.5°, the ANB angle grows smaller.

6.1.1.1 With *horizontal growth tendencies*, this phase of growth has an effect in the sagittal plane. The lower incisors may become more upright, or a shortage of space may develop in the region of the lower incisors, resulting in tertiary crowding (Fig. 146). If incisal overjet is minimal and the overbite deep, extended retention or at least follow-up until growth is complete are indicated with this growth type. Fine adjustment of incisor occlusion by selective grinding is definitely contra-indicated before growth is complete in these cases (Fig. 147). This final opportunity for correction should be taken only when further growth changes will no longer affect the result.

146

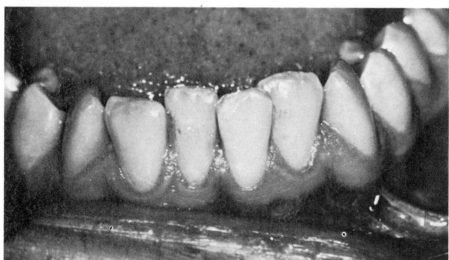

Fig. 146. Tertiary crowding.

6.1.1.2 With *vertical growth tendencies*, the final growth phase affects relationships in the anteriocaudal direction and does not influence incisor occlusion, which may therefore be adjusted on conclusion of treatment. It is not usually necessary to stabilise the lower front region by extended retention.

6.1.2 Mesial Inclination of Upper Sixth-Year Molars

This is 7° on average, with mesial migration. It arises through adaptation of the dentition to forward re-location of the mandible. Final stability depends on good interdigitation of the sixth-year molars at the end of the growth period. A Class I molar relationship is not in itself sufficient for good occlusion, and contact between the distobuccal cusps of the upper sixth and the mesiobuccal cusps of the lower second molar is also required for stability (Fig. 148; Andrews). With a Class I occlusion, this contact is obtained only through mesial inclination of the upper first molars.

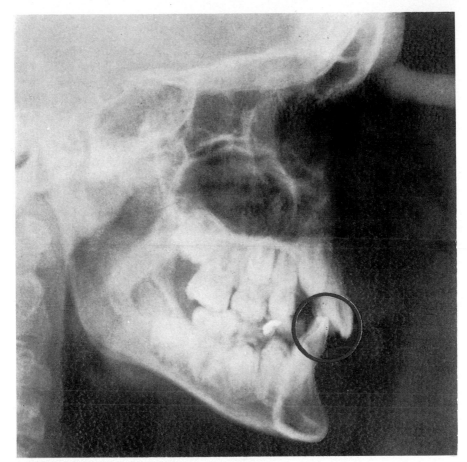

Fig. 147. Selective grinding of incisors is contra-indicated for horizontal growth types before growth has ceased.

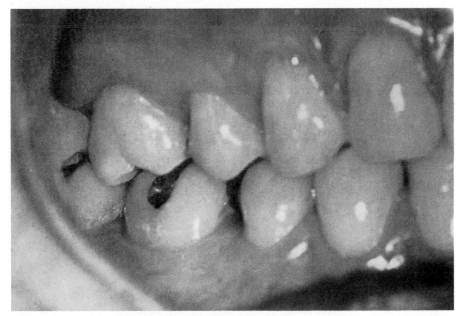

Fig. 148. Mesial tilt of 6th-year molars in the upper dental arch. Class I occlusion.

6.1.3 Final Adjustment of Occlusion

The exact relationship of the molars is determined by the final growth phase. This final adjustment is called the 'occlusal phenomenon'. The changes are due to vertical growth, especially in the condylar region. Occlusal migration of upper (1.25 mm on average) and lower molars (1 mm on average) is observed.

6.1.3.1   In horizontal growth types these changes may cause a slight opening of bite, without prejudice to the stability of treatment results.

6.1.3.2   In vertical growth types, showing minimal overbite, a slight open bite may develop during this final growth phase, and retrognathism may be enhanced (Fig. 149). Extended retention or at least follow-up observation will be required in these cases. Selective grinding is permissible only after the active growth period, to achieve a good molar relationship at a time when growth changes will no longer affect it.

149

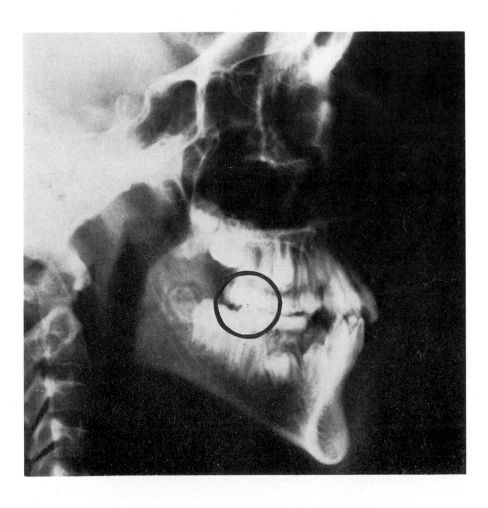

Fig. 149. Selective grinding to correct malocclusion in the molar region is contra-indicated before growth has ceased in vertical growth types.

7 Holdaway Growth Prediction

The Holdaway method holds a special position among methods of prediction. It is based on accurate construction related to reference points, but also permits individual peculiarities to be taken into account for rate of growth, direction of growth, and treatment principles. In planning, one can assess the different possibilities, depending on growth rate and treatment principles, and thus 'visualise' certain treatment objectives. Holdaway actually refers to his method as 'visualised treatment objective'.

An attractive feature of the method is its flexibility and the fact that it does not lay down treatment procedures. The orthodontist is still free to make his own decisions. We have tested the method and, in view of the above advantages, included it in our treatment programme. It enables us to make a dynamic assessment of facial morphology in many cases, and also serves as a guide in the choice of treatment principles.

7.1 The Twelve Stages of the Holdaway Analysis

To demonstrate a two-year prediction of growth, the separate stages of VTO (visualised treatment objectives) are described below. Holdaway distinguishes 12 phases in the analysis.

(1) First, the fronto-nasal area and SN and NA lines are traced on a sheet of acetate film. Growth prediction is based on changes in SN (Fig. 150).

The SNA angle may be taken to be constant for short-term prediction. According to Holdaway it probably changes by 1° in 5 years. A concomitant change in NA will therefore also serve to determine maxillary growth.

(2) Superimposing on line SN, the VTO is moved 1.5 mm along SN, relative to the original tracing. This corresponds to an annual growth of ¾ mm. In this position, the sella is drawn in, and taking into account the treatment principles, the Y axis. In most cases Holdaway opens the SN-Gn angle (Y axis) by 1–2° (Fig. 151).

We introduced a modification to the effect that the Y axis was opened by 1–2° if there was distalisation, left in its original position with activator therapy, and slightly closed with extraction therapy.

(3) Superimposing the 'VTO' Y axis on the original Y axis and using the Y axis as a growth parameter, the mandible is related downwards and forward to SN.

This determines anterior face height and the anterior position of the mandible.

The two Y axes are superimposed and the VTO is moved upward. The amount of movement should be equal to three times the amount of growth expressed previously in the fronto-nasal area (in the present case by 4.5 mm). Now the anterior portion of the mandible including the symphysis, border and Go-Gn (MP) line are drawn, and also the soft tissue chin, eliminating any hypertonicity in the mentalis (Fig. 152).

(4) Horizontal growth of the mandible is outlined by moving forward along the Go-Gn line. The posterior position of the mandible and ascending ramus are drawn when the two sellae lie in the same vertical plane (Fig. 153).

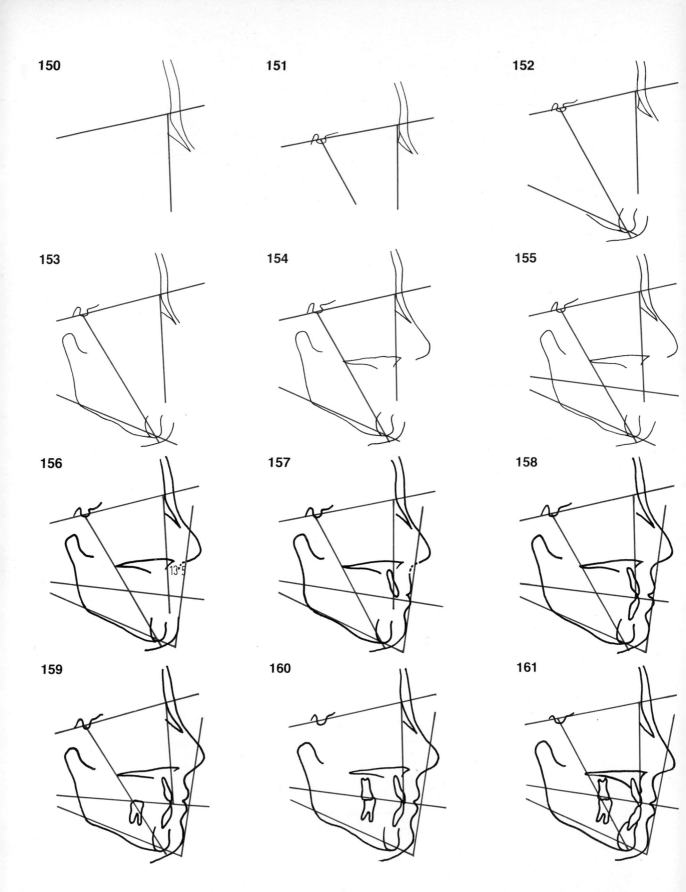

Figs. 150–155.   Holdaway stages 1–6.

Figs. 156–161.   Holdaway stages 7–12.

162

(5) On the assumption that facial growth may be divided into three sections between nasion and menton, and that the section between nasion and maxilla represents one-third of the total face height, one now proceeds to determine the vertical position of the maxilla.

The two NA lines are superimposed; 40% of total growth will lie above the SN line, 60% below Go-Gn.

The maxilla is drawn in, then point A is estimated, depending on the treatment mechanics and the nose, taking into account 1 mm of growth per annum (Fig. 154).

(6) Superimpose, with the two NA lines superimposed and the growth increase distributed so that 50% is above the maxilla, and 50% below the mandible (Fig. 155). Now draw the occlusal plane, it should lie 3 mm below the lip base.

(7) At this stage, one of the most important aspects of the VTO, the extent of repositioning of the upper incisors is determined; it serves as a guide to draw the soft tissue profile between nose and chin.

Soft tissue thickness between point A and lip profile remains unchanged. Its reposition is determined only by the new position of point A.

The structures along the maxillary base are superimposed; the soft tissue thickness taken from the original is drawn in anterior to the new point A.

The upper point for constructing the H line lies 3–7 mm anterior to the new lip profile, in the region of subnasale.

The H line is drawn from this point to the most anterior soft tissue point on the chin (Fig. 156).

(8) Relocate the upper incisors – depending on treatment principles – to allow the upper lip to rest exactly on to the H line, to create the desired aesthetic effect.

The upper lip will not follow the upper incisors until lip strain has been eliminated. The lip is free from strain when the lip thickness anterior to the incisors is within 1 mm of tissue thickness anterior to the A point.

The upper incisors are moved back by the distance to which the upper lip lies anterior to the H line plus the extent of lip tension determined by the above method, and vertically aligned to the occlusal plane.

The profile of the mouth is drawn in, with the upper lip on the H line, and the lower lip 0.5 mm anterior to the H line (Fig. 157).

(9) Superimposing the symphysis and Go-Gn line on both tracings, the lower incisors are drawn in relation to the upper incisors (Fig. 158).

(10) The lower molars are drawn, taking into account extraction and available space, with the drawings superimposed as before (Fig. 159).

(11) The upper molars are drawn, in neutral relationship (Fig. 160).

(12) At the final stage the construction is completed in the region of point A, the palate, and the symphysis (Fig. 161).

Our follow-up studies have shown that, with VTO, growth is more easily predictable in the horizontal direction, whilst vertical relationships and dento-alveolar movement were less well demonstrated.

Further modifications relating to annual growth rates, more detailed consideration of the direction of growth and the methods of treatment employed, may improve the reliability of prediction.

Cephalometric Radiography in Treatment Planning

Effective treatment planning depends on accurate diagnosis. This requires objective, relevant and accurate information, data and analyses. The criteria used should cover the whole orofacial region, yet they must also be selective. The key facts need to be considered in conjunction. Accessory details that are only of secondary importance for decisions to be made and the action to be taken, should be ignored.

Individual data need to be selectively assessed for their significance relative to the total course of treatment, so that unexpected reactions may be registered in good time. This procedure may be designated a continuous diagnostic process.

Cephalometric radiography is just one link in the complex of data collection. Its relative value in providing information for overall planning will vary from case to case, depending on the nature of the anomaly, the age of the patient, and the possible forms of treatment. Cephalometric radiography is not a once-only investigation, but needs to be repeated in the course of treatment as part of the continuous diagnostic process.

With regard to treatment, accurate planning enables:

(a) Application of the simplest and most effective form of treatment in each case.

(b) Selection not of the patient for the method, but of the method for the patient, i.e. the indication and contra-indication of different methods is established.

(c) Differential diagnosis to establish indication for various fixed or removable appliances, or for combined methods of treatment.

As an example, let us consider the most widely seen anomaly, a Class II$_1$ occlusal relationship.

1 The Role of Cephalometric Radiography in Treatment for Class II$_1$ Patients

Before proceeding to treat this anomaly (which is a collective term, and not a particular condition), a number of differential diagnostic steps have to be taken. Not only may the anomaly take many different forms, but the methods of treatment available to us – and these need to be considered in treatment planning – have changed with the times.

The different theories may be summed up as follows:

(1) Only tooth movement and dento-alveolar changes are possible.

(2) Orthodontic techniques may be effectively used to stimulate bone growth.

(3) It is possible only to bring out the individual potential for optimum growth, as already laid down genetically.

(4) Direction of growth may be changed.

(5) Orthodontic techniques can be used to change the time pattern of growth.

(6) It is possible to inhibit growth in the mid-face region.

The term Class II₁ malocclusion covers a wide range of dysgnathic conditions, and the form of treatment to be chosen will depend on the nature of the anomaly and the developmental stage of the stomatognathic system. Tooth movement in the dento-alveolar region is also possible after cessation of growth. Stimulation of bone growth, encouragement of growth potential, and changes in direction of growth cannot be contemplated after this point in time.

The time pattern of growth changes and the sequence of tooth eruption can be influenced only in mixed dentition. Guidance or inhibition of sutural growth in the mid-face region can be effected only during active growth.

The transitional dentition stage nevertheless offers the best opportunity for Class II₁ therapy.

1.1 Localisation of the Malocclusion

The key question in deciding on a course of treatment is the localisation of the anomaly within the facial skeleton. This is considered at four levels.

(1) Level one is the occlusal situation. This may be changed at any time, by minor orthodontic procedures or selective grinding.

(2) Level two is the relationship of the teeth to the periodontium. Treatment procedures in this area are indicated with dento-alveolar anomalies, or if compensation of a skeletal malocclusion in the dento-alveolar region is required. At this level, effective measures may be taken even after cessation of growth.

(3) The third level is that of the facial sutures and temporo-mandibular joints. At this level, effective treatment is possible only during active phases of growth. In cases of skeletal malocclusion, growth may be inhibited or stimulated by headgear or activator therapy. Once growth has ceased, changes in skeletal relationship can be effected only through surgical measures.

(4) The fourth level, that of the synchondroses and cranial sutures, cannot be influenced by orthodontic therapy.

Localisation of the malocclusion, taking into account the periods of active growth still to come, permits the decision to be made as to whether treatment should be causal or compensatory. Dento-alveolar Class II relationships usually permit causal rehabilitation. With skeletal Class II relationships, on the other hand, this is possible only during active growth, on the condition that the direction of growth is also favourable.

Cephalometric radiography provides the data for diagnostic differentiation between skeletal and dento-alveolar Class II anomalies. If the anomaly is skeletal the ANB angle is large, due to the SNB angle being too small and/or the SNA angle too large. With a dento-alveolar Class II anomaly, the upper incisors lie anterior to the NPog line, with the lower incisors frequently situated behind this line; protrusion is frequently seen in the maxilla, and very upright incisors in the mandible. The skeletal relationships are balanced. The history will often reveal dysfunction or early loss of primary teeth.

1.2 Functional Assessment of Class II Occlusion

Cephalometric radiography will provide valuable additional information in functional analysis.

1.2.1 Relationship of Rest to Occlusal Position

This can be accurately recorded and analysed by radiography. The following variations may be found.

1.2.1.1 The movement of the mandible is hinge-like as it changes from the rest to the occlusal position, i.e. functional and morphological relationships are in accord, the anomaly shows functional balance with no translocation. Intermaxillary relationships and the rest position can only be changed during active growth, if at all.

1.2.1.2 The mandible moves forward as it changes from the rest to the occlusal position. The functional disorder is more serious than assessment of the occlusal position would suggest. Translocation results in forward sliding of the mandible, and the full extent of the anomaly can only be assessed once this has been eliminated. The prognosis is poor with anterior displacement of the mandible, the only possible form of correction being distalisation of the upper teeth.

1.2.1.3 The mandible moves backwards as it changes from the rest to the occlusal position. Its anterior position at rest shows a Class I relationship, retrusion occurring through translocation. This may arise not only through abnormal contacts in the intercuspidation, but also through incisor guidance with deep overbite. Adequate correction may be achieved by eliminating the translocation.

1.2.2 Assessment of Lip Configuration in Relation to Incisor Relationship and Angulation (Fig. 162a, b; 163a, b)

The relationship of upper and lower incisors to the lower lip may be shown in the radiograph. Depending on the direction of loading, the upper incisors may be tipped labially through palatal pressure and/or the lower incisors lingually. Lip dysfunction will have much more serious consequences with a Class II skeletal relationship – because of the unfavourable relationship of the maxillary and mandibular bases – than would be the case with an orthognathic skeletal relationship.

1.2.3 Assessment of Tongue Position and Consequences of Tongue Dysfunction

The position of the tongue may be demonstrated radiographically. With a flat, retracted tongue the prognosis for forward positioning of the mandible is poor. Depending on cranial relationships, tongue dysfunction will have different effects in a Class II relationship. With a horizontal growth pattern, tongue thrust results in bialveolar protrusion; with vertical growth pattern, it causes very upright positioning of the lower incisors (Fig. 164, 165).

1.2.4 Assessment of Upper Airway Patency

Enlarged adenoids may be distinguished in the radiograph. A flat tongue and vertical lip incompetence are further symptoms characteristically seen with oral breathing (Fig. 166a, b).

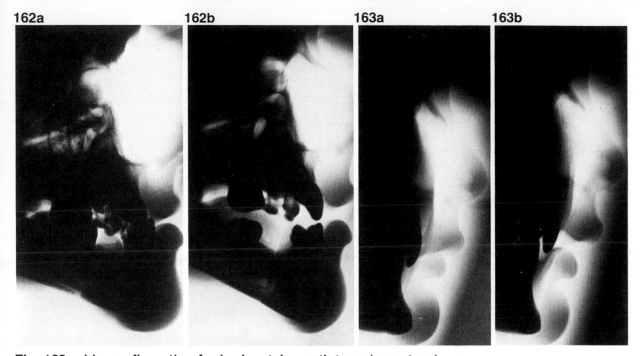

Fig. 163. Lip configuration for horizontal growth type, in occlusal (a) and rest position (b) of the mandible.

Fig. 162. Lip configuration for vertical growth type, in occlusal (a) and rest position (b) of the mandible.

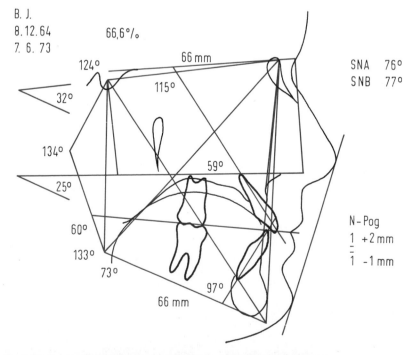

Fig. 164. Tracing from radiograph of a patient with tongue thrust, horizontal growth type. Tongue thrust has produced a bialveolar protrusion. Relation of posterior to anterior face height 66.6%, protrusion of upper and lower incisors.

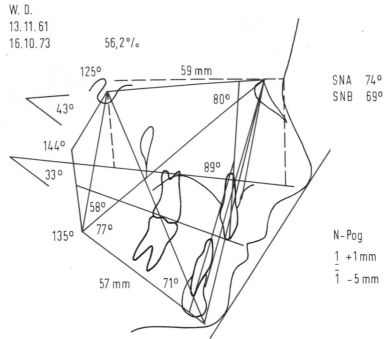

W. D.
13.11.61
16.10.73   56,2°/o

125°   59 mm
43°
80°   SNA 74°
SNB 69°
144°
33°   89°

58°
135° 77°   N-Pog

57 mm   71°   1 +1mm
                      ─
                      1 -5mm

Fig. 165. Tracing from radiograph of patient with vertical growth trend and tongue thrust. Tongue thrust has given rise to upright position of incisors, mainly in the mandible. Relation of posterior to anterior face height 56%, inclination of long axis of lower incisors relative to MP 71°.

166a   166b

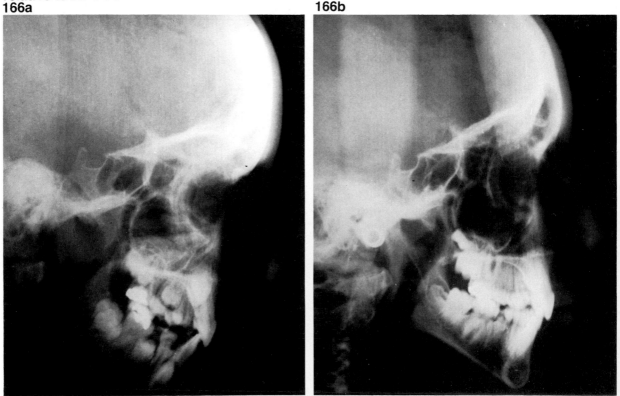

Fig. 166. Assessment of adenoids in the radiograph. (a) Large adenoids, patency of upper respiratory passages reduced. (b) The same patient after adenoidectomy.

1.3 Growth Direction

For treatment planning, it is essential to determine the direction of growth.

If the growth type is horizontal, correction of antero-posterior jaw relationship usually presents no difficulties, whilst that of deep bite is difficult, and will no longer be possible following extraction of the premolars.

If the growth type is vertical, opening the bite usually presents no problem, but correction of the antero-posterior dental arch relationship is frequently not possible. Good results may be obtained following extraction of the premolars.

1.4 Growth Potential

Therapeutic correction of the occlusion is partly contingent on phases of active growth. One problem of diagnosis is determination of prospective growth. If the mandible is too small in cases of Class II malocclusion in mixed dentition, growth may be expected to be quite considerable. A well developed mandible in a posterior position must be considered to offer poor prospects for successful correction of Class II malocclusions, except in cases with translocation. In assessment, distinction must always be made between position and size, and it is for this reason that not only angles but also dimensions are determined.

1.5 Aetiological Assessment

When the anomaly has been localised within the facial skeleton, and functional relationships have been determined, it is possible to draw certain conclusions as to the cause of the malocclusion. With skeletal Class II anomalies the causal factor is hereditary. Dysfunction on the other hand will give rise to malocclusions localisable to the dento-alveolar region.

2 Detailed Treatment Plan

Evaluation and assessment being complete, it is now necessary to decide on the plan of treatment.

During the mixed dentition period Class II occlusions may be treated as follows:

(1) Elimination of dysfunction by inhibitional therapy.

(2) Anterior positioning of the mandible with functional appliances.

(3) Movement distally in the upper jaw with headgear therapy.

(4) A combination of (1) to (3).

2.1 Elimination of Dysfunction

Adverse habits may be treated by inhibition or the use of a screen (the Fränkel function corrector is an appliance of this type). If the cause of the anomaly is a functional disorder (e.g. consequence of a sucking habit), elimination of the causal factor should enable further development to follow a normal course. Tongue thrust or lip sucking needs to be eliminated and function restored to normal if optimum development of the dentition is to be ensured. A pre-condition for successful treatment in these cases is that endogenous development must follow normal trends. Cephalometric radiography plays a key role in the differential diagnosis. If the history and clinical and functional analysis suggest dysfunction as the causal factor in the anomaly, radiography will be needed to confirm the tentative diagnosis. The influence of abnormal muscle pressures may be localised in the dento-alveolar region. If there should also be a skeletal component, this will be developmental in origin and can be influenced by inhibitory treatment only indirectly, at the beginning of the mixed dentition period at the latest. Inhibition therapy will only inhibit the functional factor, permitting unrestricted growth to the patient's inherent potential.

The effects of dysfunction are entirely limited to the dento-alveolar region, as is evident from numerous clinical and experimental studies. Hypoglossia provides an excellent illustration of this. The condition will cause inhibition of growth, but only in the dento-alveolar region.

A male patient aged 35 presented with severe malocclusion due to hypoglossia. Cephalometric radiography revealed a horizontal growth type, a small gonial angle, and normally developed maxillary and mandibular bases. Severe abnormality was however found in the dento-alveolar relationship of the anterior teeth. The upper incisors were 8 mm anterior to the NPog line, with their long axis at an angle of 117° to the SN plane. The lower incisors were 16 mm posterior to the NPog line, and very upright, at 74° to the MP (Fig. 167a, b; 168a, b).

Inhibitional therapy, designed to restore abnormal function to normal, is a causal form of treatment, and can be effectively used only during the phase of active growth. It will be most effective during the eruption of the permanent incisors, when not only bone growth but also the eruption potential are fully utilisable, and it is possible to influence development in the region of the facial skeleton.

A 6-year-old boy (B.N.) presented with marked Class II₁ malocclusion and adverse lip pressures after eruption of the lower incisors (Fig. 169a, b). The anomaly was very marked for such an early age, with a skeletal and a dento-alveolar component as well as severe dysfunction. Early treatment, during the changing of the incisors, was indicated. It is still possible at this stage of development to eliminate the dysfunction and normalise function, and thus also achieve a positive change in skeletal development. When all the incisors have erupted, this possibility generally ceases to exist.

The patient showed marked horizontal growth tendencies, the relationship of posterior to anterior face height being 67%. Mid-face development was considerable, with an SNA angle of 81.5°. The mandibular base was retrognathic, with SNB 74.5°, and too short (−8 mm). The basal discrepancy of the ANB angles was 7°. The upper deciduous incisors were 9 mm anterior to the NPog line, the lower permanent incisors 4.5 mm posterior to it.

Inhibitional therapy was initiated. A screen was made to fit the vestibule, and this was designed not only to eliminate the dysfunction, but also to permit forward movement of the mandible and inhibit growth in the upper apical region.

2.1.1   Principles of Inhibition Therapy

At this point, reference may be made to some of the principles of inhibition or screening therapy. This approach is governed by functional considerations.

2.1.1.1   Function also implies the application of mechanical force exerting strain. If the mechanical stress has a fixed direction, a change is produced in the dynamic balance and hence in bone structure.

The functional forces applied produce changes in alveolar bone, with tissue adaptation occurring secondarily. The concepts on which inhibition therapy is based may be summarised as follows:

(a) Function has a considerable influence on structure.

(b) A natural function will produce a natural structure.

(c) An unnatural function will produce an unnatural structure.

(d) Changes in function will also lead to changes in structure.

2.1.1.2   On the other hand it must be stressed that, like all biological functions, tissues have a common property, i.e. a certain ability to adhere to a developmental trend that is phylo-genetically predetermined.

Negative external factors are thus countered by heredity. If the hereditary disposition is a normal one, the developmental trend of the stomatognathic system will also be normal.

The effects of external factors are under certain conditions counterbalanced by hereditary factors. The pre-condition for achieving such a balance is elimination of unfavourable external factors during the early stages of development. The early exclusion of harmful exogenic factors can enable normal development of the dentition to take place.

The principle of this form of screening is that the situation normalises itself once external factors liable to interfere with normal development have been eliminated. The pre-conditions for this are:

(a) A normal endogenous development trend.

(b) Causal intervention has to be applied at an early stage, when the masticatory system still has growth potential.

The therapy is called inhibitory because reflexes of unphysiological origin are inhibited and normal development is encouraged. This form of treatment does not enable one to move teeth or guide development in the maxilla or mandible. It merely excludes malfunction to permit normal development, i.e. one is simulating spontaneous correction. The treatment is physiological and causal, with no risk of tissue damage or relapse; we are thus breaking the unnatural reflex sequence at one point, and enabling the rehabilitation of natural reflexes.

2.1.1.3   The requirements for these applicances, which do not involve the application of force, but merely the elimination of pressure, are as follows:

(a) They are designed to eliminate unnatural function.

(b) They must not prevent the tissue from returning to its normal configuration.

(c) They should replace the original signal, the stimulus.

2.1.1.4   The vestibular screen indicated in the case of patient B.N. had to be constructed, according to specific principles, to meet the requirements outlined above (Fig. 170a, b, c).

167a

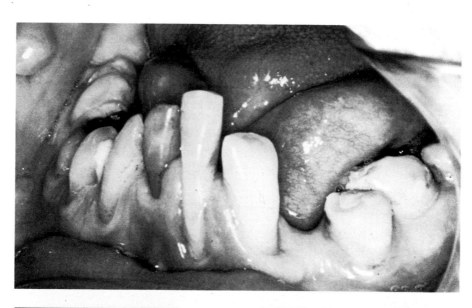

167b

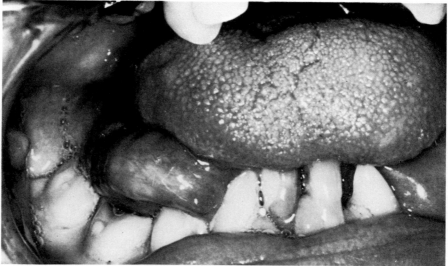

Fig. 167.   Male patient aged 35 with hypoglossia. (a) Floor of mouth clearly visible, (b) patient with maximum protrusion of tongue.

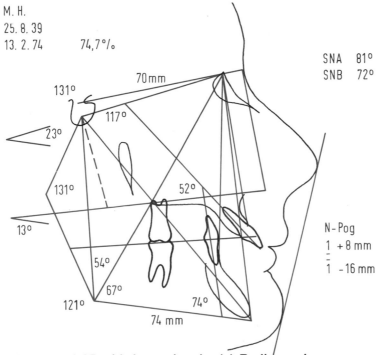

M. H.
25. 8. 39
13. 2. 74   74,7 %

131°
23°
117°
131°
13°
52°
54°
67°
121°
74°
74 mm
70 mm

SNA 81°
SNB 72°

N - Pog
1 + 8 mm
1 - 16 mm

Fig. 168. Male patient aged 35 with hypoglossia. (a) Radiograph, (b) tracing.

173

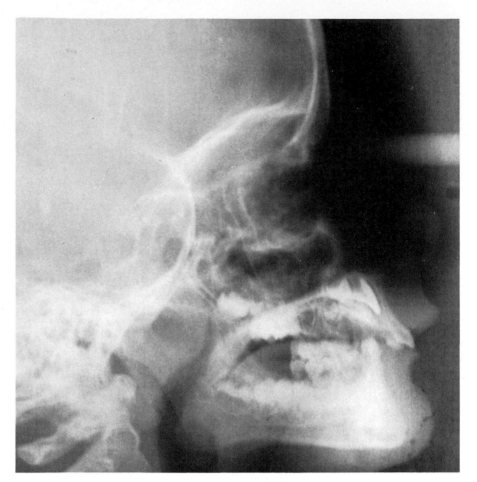

B. N.
24. 5. 70

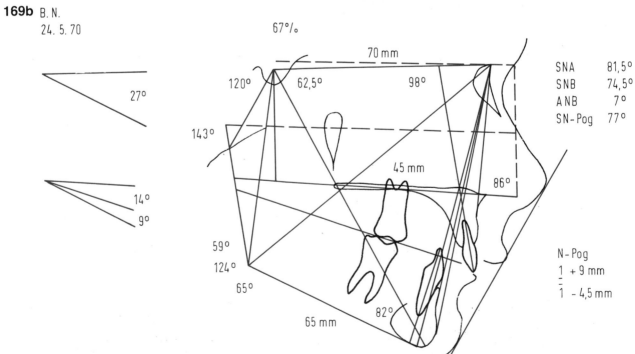

67‰

70 mm

120°   62,5°   98°

143°

45 mm

86°

59°

124°

65°

82°

65 mm

27°

14°
9°

SNA   81,5°
SNB   74,5°
ANB   7°
SN-Pog 77°

N-Pog
$\underline{1}$ + 9 mm
$\bar{\underline{1}}$ - 4,5 mm

Fig. 169.   Patient B.N., before treatment. (a) Radiograph, (b) tracing.

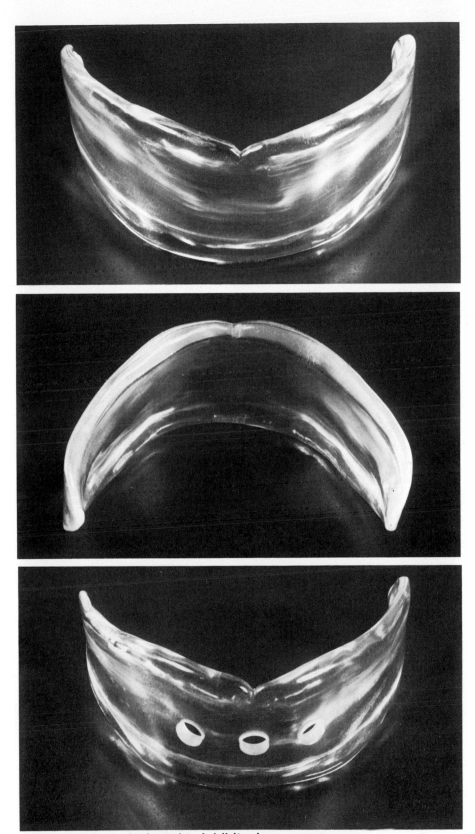

Fig. 170.   Vestibular screen designed to inhibit adverse pressures.
(a) Anterior view, (b) inner surface of the appliance, (c) appliance
with holes.

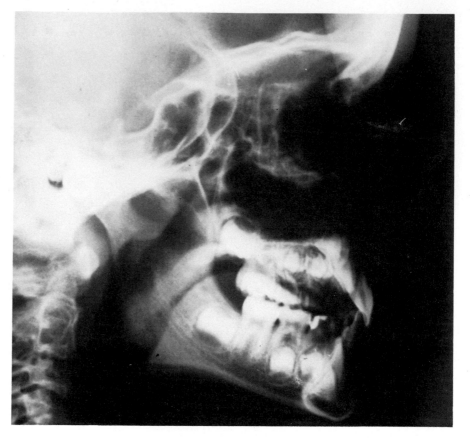

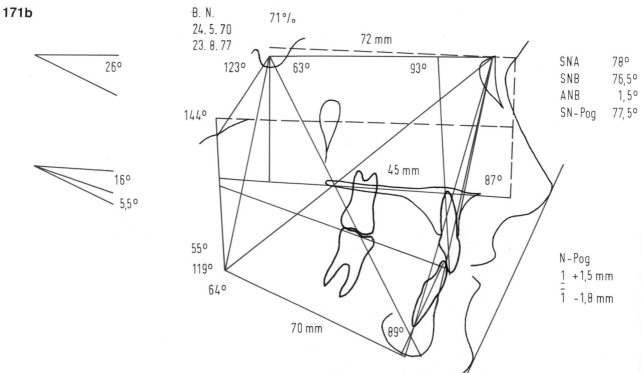

26°

16°
5,5°

B. N.
24. 5. 70
23. 8. 77

71%

72 mm

123°   63°   93°

144°

45 mm   87°

55°
119°

64°

70 mm   89°

SNA   78°
SNB   76,5°
ANB   1,5°
SN-Pog   77,5°

N-Pog
$\frac{1}{1}$ +1,5 mm
$\frac{1}{1}$ −1,8 mm

Fig. 171. Patient B.N., after 12 months treatment. (a) Radiograph,
(b) tracing.

The screen is made in revised working bite, does not come in contact with the teeth, and extends throughout the vestibule, from the upper to the lower muco-labial fold and posteriorly as far as the last molars. Direct contact with the mucous membrane exists only in the region of the upper mucolabial fold. The teeth on the plaster model were coated with wax before the screen was constructed on the model, to prevent direct contact.

After one year's treatment with the vestibular plate, extensive changes were noted in the skeletal and alveolar regions (Fig. 171a, b). The ANB angle had been reduced to 1.5°, due to a reduction in SNA to 78°, whilst SNB had increased to 76.5°. Forward movement of the mandible had occurred in conjunction with a 5 mm increase in its length. The age-related increment would have been no more than 2 mm. No growth changes were noted in the area of the maxillary base. Vertical growth showed a considerable overall increase amounting to 7 mm in posterior face height (5 mm above the average rate) and 8 mm in anterior face height (also 5 mm above the average). The horizontal growth tendency had increased (to 71%), the incisor relationship become normal, with the upper incisors now 1.5 mm anterior and the lower incisor 1.8 mm posterior to the NPog line.

The appliance was used during a phase of active growth. It eliminated factors inhibiting mandibular growth, and inhibited growth in the maxillary region. It would not have been possible to achieve the 5.5° reduction in ANB angle with such simple means at a later stage of development.

2.1.2 Indication of Inhibition Therapy

This form of treatment is frequently indicated in both primary and mixed dentition.

2.1.2.1   With primary dentition, it may be used:

(a) For all acquired anomalies arising through malfunction.

(b) For disorders of speech, swallowing and breathing that are of peripheral origin.

(c) As a preliminary form of treatment where activator therapy is to follow.

(d) For follow-up treatment of habitual mouth breathing after adenectomy.

2.1.2.2   Indication in Mixed Dentition

With mixed dentition, inhibition therapy will not usually be adequate as the sole form of treatment, and it will be necessary to use the method in conjunction with others.

2.1.2.2.1   Inhibition therapy as the only form of treatment is in principle sufficient only where there is no need to alter the rest position of the mandible. In contra-distinction to the primary dentition, the range of indication is limited with this group. Only recently acquired anomalies can be considered, where no other abnormality is present apart from the consequences of dysfunction.

Very much as in the case of the primary dentition, it is enough to change the external factors to allow spontaneous correction to take place.

In these cases, inhibition therapy is causal, effective and physiological.

The results of treatment with screen appliances are not results of treatment in the active sense. We are however making it possible for the dentition to develop in the normal way for that particular dentition.

That is the essential nature of inhibition therapy, and the method is not difficult to use. In making the diagnosis, it is however important to make an accurate clinical assessment, and here functional analysis and cephalometric radiography are of prime importance in determining the indication. If development is following a normal pattern and no changes are required in the rest position, inhibition therapy may be expected to give good results. If development is not along normal lines, our efforts to change exogenic factors are in vain. We are then not dealing with normal development, but one that is normal for that particular dentition only, and, according to our concepts, abnormal.

2.1.2.2.2 In mixed dentition, inhibition therapy is very frequently indicated in conjunction with another form of treatment:

(a) In cases where inhibition therapy corrects the part of the anomaly that has been caused by dysfunction. Any anomaly still persisting after such preliminary treatment may be considered due to heredity.

Treatment is then continued with active therapy, and after preliminary inhibition therapy this can give good results.

Inhibition therapy is frequently combined with functional orthodontic therapy, where elimination of the dysfunction and its sequelae is followed by functional appliance treatment. This approach is indicated particularly where dysfunction needs to be eliminated before functional orthodontic therapy is initiated, or for children who because of lack of tone in the circumoral musculature have difficulty in getting used to a functional appliance.

In the course of such preliminary treatment, one will often observe a considerable change in intermaxillary relationships.

(b) The usual form of functional orthodontic therapy may also be combined with concurrent inhibition therapy; if an activator is worn at night, for example, harmful external factors can be eliminated during the day by use of a lower lip or tongue screen.

(c) Inhibition therapy is also indicated as a preliminary to activator therapy in cases of habitual mouth breathing with lip incompetence.

We have found that the resting position of the tongue takes two forms:

Type 1: The dorsum is flat, the tongue extends over the floor of the mouth within the lower dental arch. This tongue position is seen with prognathism and where mouth breathing is nasal in origin, occurring in conjunction with massively enlarged adenoids.

Type 2: Tongue retracted, with dorsum curving to form an arch. The tip of the tongue is on the line joining the premolars or sixth-year molars.

The vestibular screen is effective with the type 2 tongue position. Following insertion of the screen, the tongue achieves a higher position and hence contact with the soft palate.

In establishing the indication of inhibition therapy, cephalometric radiography may be used to support clinical assessment and functional analysis.

2.1.2.3 The Role of Cephalometric Radiography in Establishing the Indication for Inhibition Therapy

Cephalometric radiography makes it possible to judge whether if after elimination of the dysfunction the growth trend is likely to be normal. The principal signs required to establish the indication may be summarised as follows:

(a) Differential diagnosis of primary and secondary tongue dysfunction. With primary tongue dysfunction, the anomaly is located in the dento-alveolar region. The SN-MeGo angle, the angle of the base plane, the angle between the occlusal and mandibular planes, is small, with the growth type more horizontal. The malocclusion has been caused by tongue dysfunction. Secondary tongue dysfunction consists of adaptation in the tongue function to a skeletal open bite. The above-mentioned angles are large, with growth direction vertical.

(b) Differential diagnosis of overjet due to lip dysfunction and overjet arising from a discrepancy between the maxillary bases.

With overjet due to lip dysfunction, skeletal relations are within normal range (ANB angle). The upper incisors are tipped labially, and the lower lingually. The lower incisors lie behind the NPog line. If the overjet is due to skeletal discrepancy, the ANB angle is large, the lower incisors frequently lie anterior to the NPog line, and the lip dysfunction may be secondary, due to adaptation to the undesirable skeletal relationship.

Inhibition therapy is indicated only with the first group.

2.1.3.1 Lower Lip Screen

If a Class II/1 malocclusion in the mixed dentition with marked overjet and lip dysfunction is to be corrected, a combination of activator or perhaps also headgear therapy and a lower lip screen will frequently be the method of choice. A lower lip screen is in fact the lower half of a vestibular screen. It is positioned in the region of the lower alveolar process and extends to the level of the incisal third of the lower teeth. Contact with the mucosa is limited to the area of the muco-labial fold, and there is no contact with the teeth. Anchorage may be achieved by using inverted Adams clasps fitted to the sixth-year molars. Apart from this, the screen does not touch the teeth, and even in closed bite there is no contact with the upper teeth (Fig. 172a, b).

The indication for a lower lip screen is based on the facial type and the angulation of the lower incisors as determined by cephalometric radiography.

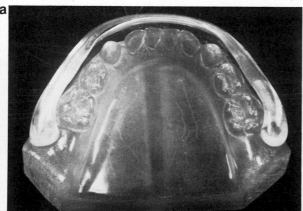 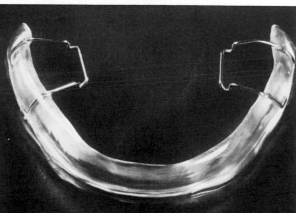

Fig. 172. Lower lip screen, (a) with deciduous teeth, (b) with inverted Adams clasps in mixed dentition.

In patients with mentalis muscle dysfunction, lower lip screen therapy aims to achieve a direct effect on the lower lip. The use of the screen does however cause a shift in the balance of the orofacial system. Our own palatographic studies have shown that a lower lip screen will have a direct effect on the tongue. A change in functional balance in the labial region will lead to a forward displacement of the tongue (Fig. 173a-d). Labial tilt of the lower incisors will also be noted. Headgear therapy will produce similar side effects.

173a

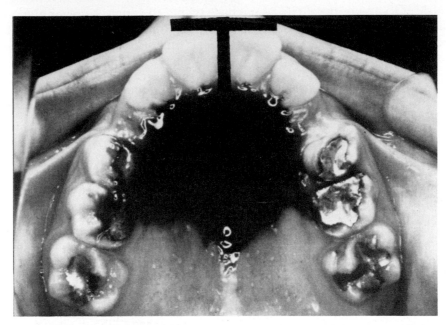

173b

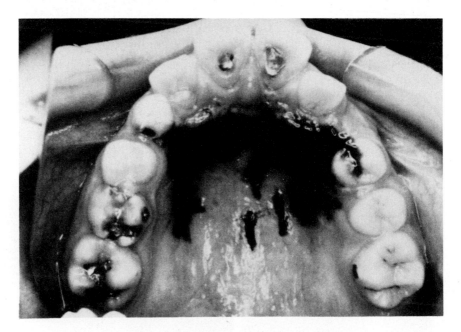

Fig. 173. Palatographic study of the tongue. (a) Distance from the tip of the tongue to the upper incisors, (b) palatogram of a patient without (c) and with lower lip screen, (d) lower lip screen in the mouth.

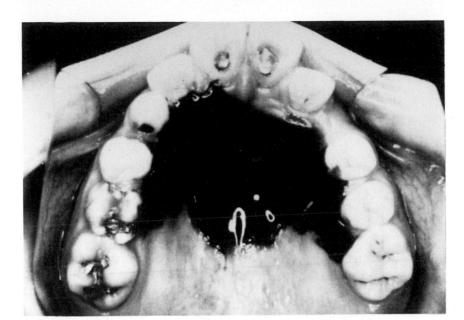

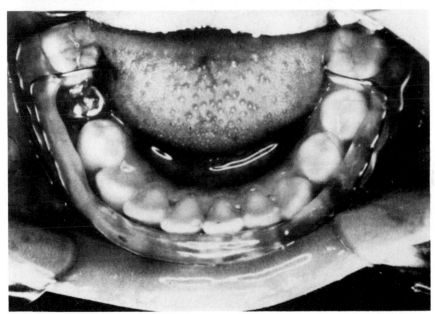

(a) A vertical growth type shows predisposition for visceral swallowing.

Tongue thrust is frequently seen in this group, and the thrust is quite marked, with considerable contraction of the circumoral musculature. The tongue lies flat, protruding interdentally. Marked contraction of the mentalis muscle causes the anterior segments of the lower arch to be retro-inclined, giving a very upright position.

(b) With the horizontal growth type, the tip of the tongue does not protrude to the same extent during thrust, and presses against the upper and lower dental arches. As a result, one often sees bialveolar protrusion.

It is only rarely that one notes sucking in of the lower lip with this growth type.

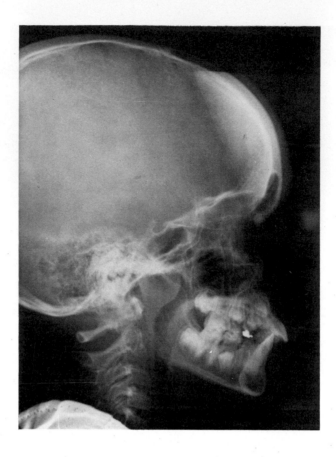

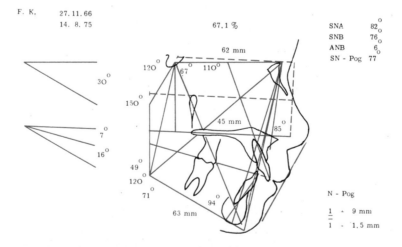

F. K.   27.11.66
          14. 8. 75

67.1 %

SNA   82°
SNB   76°
ANB   6°
SN - Pog 77°

62 mm

120°   67° 110°

30°

150°

45 mm   85

7°

16°

49°

120°

71°

94

63 mm

N - Pog

$\underline{1}$ - 9 mm
$\overline{1}$ - 1.5 mm

Fig. 174.   Nine-year-old girl (F.K.) with Class II/1 malocclusion and 110° labial tipping of upper incisors. (a) Cephalometric radiograph, (b) tracing.

The inner arch of the headgear indirectly has the effect of screening off the perioral musculature. This will inevitably cause forward displacement of the tongue.

The undesirable side effects of inhibition therapy show up early in the radiograph. The side effects due to screening of the perioral musculature were clearly demonstrable in the case of our patient F.K. (Fig. 174a, b).

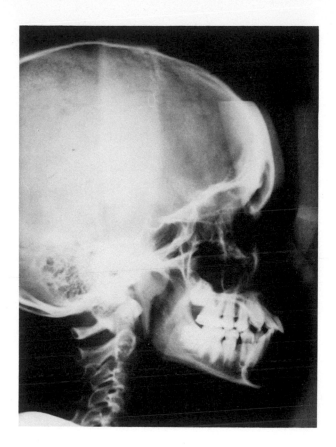

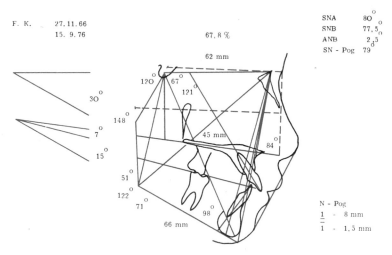

F. K.   27.11.66
15. 9. 76   67,8 %

62 mm

120° 67°
121°
30°
148°
7°
45 mm
84°
15°
51°
122°
71°
98°
66 mm

SNA   80°
SNB   77,5°
ANB   2,5°
SN - Pog 79°

N - Pog
$\underline{1}$ - 8 mm
$\overline{1}$ - 1,5 mm

Fig. 175. Patient F.K. after a year's treatment with headgear and lower lip screen. Labial tipping of upper incisors 121°. (a) Cephalometric radiograph, (b) tracing.

The patient, a 9-year-old girl, presented with a Class II₁ malocclusion, labial tilt of the upper incisors, and lip dysfunction. As the SNA angle was enlarged, treatment was initiated with headgear. In the course of this, Class I dentition was achieved in the molar region and the ANB angle reduced. Screening of the perioral musculature by the inner arch of the headgear did however cause a very marked labial tilt of the upper incisors (Fig. 175a, b).

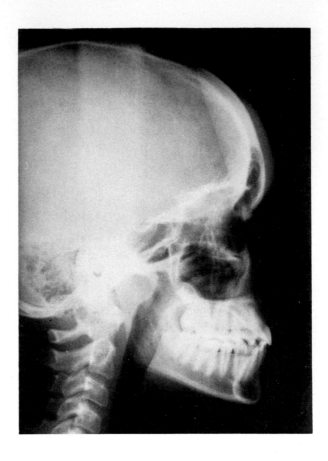

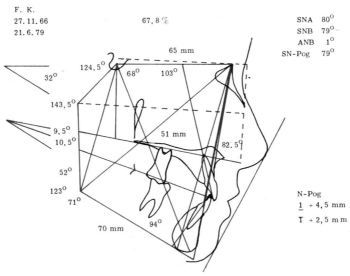

F. K.
27. 11. 66
21. 6. 79

67, 8 %

SNA 80°
SNB 79°
ANB 1°
SN-Pog 79°

124, 5°   68°   103°   65 mm

32°

143, 5°

9, 5°
10, 5°   51 mm   82, 5°

52°

123°
71°

70 mm   94°

N-Pog
1 + 4, 5 mm
I + 2, 5 mm

Fig. 176. Patient F.K. on conclusion of activator therapy. Angulation of incisors corrected. (a) Cephalometric radiograph, (b) tracing.

It required several years of activator therapy to achieve correct incisor angulation (Fig. 176a, b).

2.2 The Usefulness of Cephalometric Radiography with Functional Orthodontic Treatment

Principles of Activator Therapy

Orthodontic treatment always involves the application of force, in the form of pressure, traction, and shearing forces.

This application of force causes stresses in the tissues, with the treatment-induced changes continuing until a new state of balance is established. Methods of treatment differ in the source of the force applied.

With the activator, the force components originate in the musculature. In construction bite, the mandible is displaced from its balanced position (i.e. the rest position) and the muscle tension thus produced provides the force used in treatment.

(a) The force may be transferred to the temporomandibular joints and the sutures of the facial skeleton to encourage or inhibit growth in these areas.

(b) The dento-alveolar or parodontal action of the activator arises through transfer of the force to the teeth and alveolar processes.

The Indications for Activator Therapy with the Aid of Cephalometric Radiography

To establish the indication for activator therapy it is necessary to determine if the conditions for a forward repositioning of the mandible have been met.

2.2.1 First Condition

The first condition is that the mandible must be in a posterior position and the SNB angle small. If the mandibular base is too short, the posterior position may be assumed to be due to growth deficiency. If the mandible is well developed, translocated closure due to backward movement of the mandible may be found. The probable diagnosis based on the radiograph must be confirmed by functional assessment. A growth-conditioned posterior position can be corrected by functional orthodontic treatment during the growth phase, posterior translocated closure may also be corrected at a later age, when growth has ceased, by changing the occlusal plane.

2.2.2 Second Condition

Correction of malocclusion consisting of conventional activator therapy is possible only where the growth pattern is horizontal or at least indifferent. If the growth direction is vertical, the mandible cannot be brought forward, but only down and forward, and this will not correct the skeletal Class II relationship. The treatment prognosis is unfavourable if the ratio of posterior to anterior face height is less than 60%, the sum of posterior angles greater than 400°, or the lower gonial angle greater than 76°. If the lower incisors are very upright, correction of a Class II relationship can be supported by correcting the angle of the lower incisors. If the lower incisors show labial tilt, dento-alveolar compensation is not a possibility.

2.2.3 Third Condition

A further precondition for correction of Class II malocclusion by bringing forward the mandible is that the maxilla must be in normal position. If the mid-face is convex and the maxilla prognathic, the mandible cannot be brought forward into an unnatural prognathic position as well. An excessively large SNA angle frequently indicates the need for distal movement in the maxilla. Combined treatment is often indicated, bringing the mandible forward and effecting distal movement in the maxilla (Fig. 177).

177

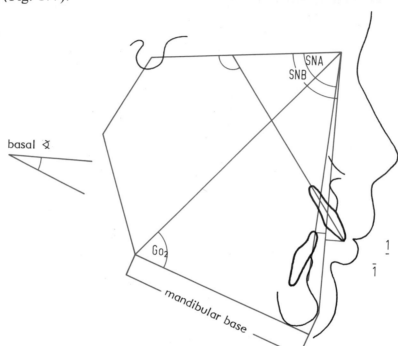

Fig. 177. Indication for activator therapy. The principal radiological criteria, diagrammatic.

2.2.4 Taking the Working Bite

Before taking the construction bite it will be necessary to determine the extent of forward and opening movement required, and whether mid-line correction is indicated. The skeletal relationship, inclination of the incisors, and direction of growth should be assessed radiographically.

As the musculature is activated when taking the construction bite, the skeletal pattern in the skull must also be taken into account. For a horizontal growth type, the construction bite is taken as follows:

(1) Maximum forward displacement in the sagittal plane until edge bite is achieved, parallel to the functional occlusal plane.

(2) In the vertical plane we stay in the range of the rest position. With the bite taken in this way, intermittent forces of the masticatory musculature are activated, and myotatic reflex activity is initiated via muscle spindles.

Activator therapy was indicated in the case of a girl aged 8 presenting with average direction of growth, retrognathic skeletal relationship, and labial inclination of the upper incisors (Fig. 178a, b). With an average direction of growth at this age, a shift towards the horizontal may be expected during subsequent years.

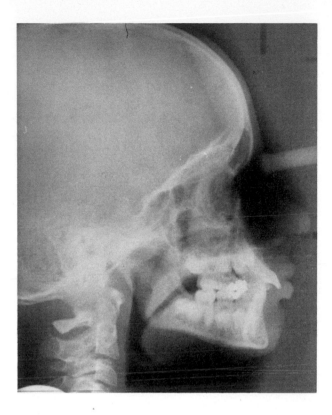

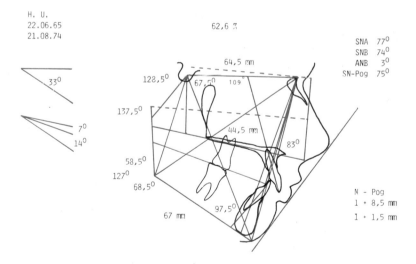

Fig. 178. Patient H.U. with retrognathic skeletal relationship, average growth trend and labial tipping of incisors. (a) Cephalometric radiograph, (b) tracing.

This is another reason why with this type of skeletal relationship activator therapy is indicated in the early mixed dentition period.

Treatment was successfully concluded within a period of 4 years. The follow-up examination shows the stability achieved, confirming the original assumption that growth would become horizontal (Fig. 179a, b).

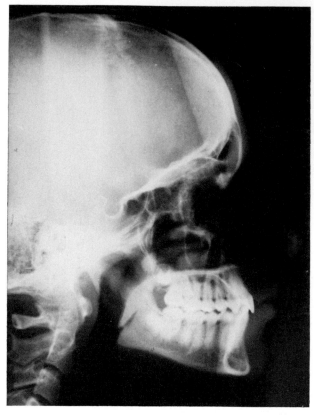

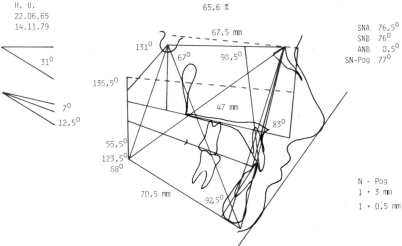

H. U.
22.06.65
14.11.79

65,6 %

67,5 mm

131°

67°

98,5°

136,5°

47 mm

83°

55,5°
123,5°
68°

70,5 mm

92,5°

31°

7°

12,5°

SNA 76,5°
SNB 76°
ANB 0,5°
SN-Pog 77°

N - Pog
1 + 3 mm

1 + 0,5 mm

Fig. 179.   Patient H.U. on conclusion of activator therapy. Horizontal relationship of facial skeleton, incisor angulation correct, growth increment in mandible 3½ mm. (a) Cephalometric radiograph, (b) tracing.

A girl aged 10 (N.G.) presented with Class II₁ malocclusion and average direction of growth (Fig. 180a–f). A small Go₂ angle did however indicate that horizontal growth tendencies were likely to develop. The maxilla was orthognathic, with an SNA angle of 81°, the mandible retrognathic, the SNB angle being 74°. The ANB angle thus was 7°. The extent of the mandible was slightly below normal. The upper incisors were tilted forward and 7.5 mm anterior to the NPog line. The position of the lower incisors, at +3 mm, was correct. Their forward angulation was extreme, however, at 108°. The mid-face was convex, with the convexity due to

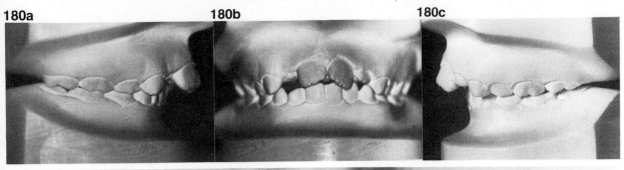

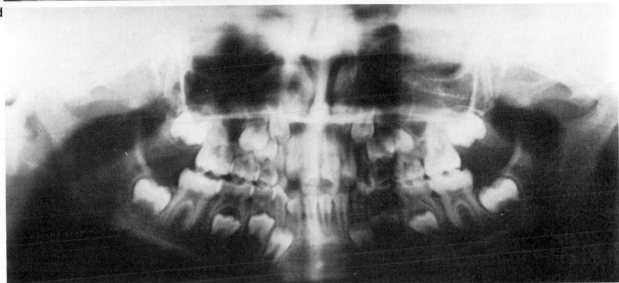

**Fig. 180.   Patient N.G., before orthodontic treatment. (a), (b), (c)
Model, (d) orthopantomogram, (e) radiograph, (f) tracing.**

an ante-inclination of 5° (90° instead of 85°).

Headgear therapy was chosen for the first stage of treatment, for the following reasons: Inhibition of growth in the mid-face region was indicated, because of the ante-inclination. A headgear with appropriate traction will not only inhibit growth potential, but also reduce ante-inclination. Correction of the Class II malocclusion by adapting the position of the mandible to the forward rotation of the maxilla was not possible. A further problem with correction of Class II malocclusion by bringing the mandible forward, was the angulation of the lower incisors. This needed correction, but bringing the incisors upright made the antero-posterior relationship worse. Dental compensation based on the lower dentition was not possible. On the contrary, after correcting lower incisor inclination, the mandible would need to be brought even further forward.

After headgear therapy, both the position of the sixth-year molars and the ante-inclination were corrected (Fig. 181a–e). An activator was then used to induce forward movement of the mandible, and the lower incisors moved to an upright position. After treatment, the ANB angle was 2°, the SNA angle had been reduced, the SNB angle enlarged. The angulation of the incisors and their position relative to the NPog line were normal. The inclination of the maxilla was now 83°. The horizontal growth tendency has increased to 65%. In the course of the last three years, an increase of 6.6 mm was noted in the length of the mandibular base, and of 4.5 mm in that of the maxilla. During the stage of headgear therapy, the increase in growth occurred not in the anterior, but rather in the posterior region, so that the distance S-S′ was reduced.

180e

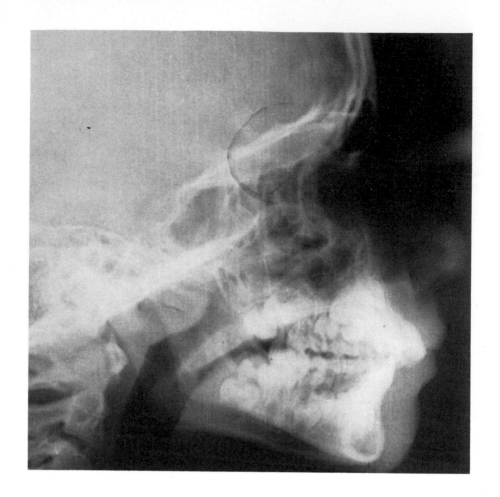

180f

N. G.
17. 7. 65
12. 11. 75

62,4 %

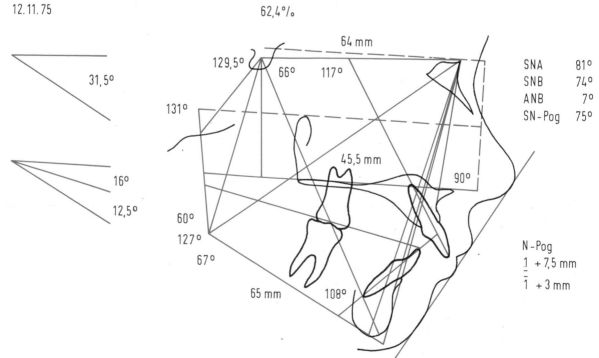

31,5°

16°

12,5°

64 mm

129,5°   66°   117°

131°

45,5 mm

90°

60°
127°

67°

65 mm   108°

SNA   81°
SNB   74°
ANB   7°
SN-Pog   75°

N-Pog
$\frac{1}{1}$ + 7,5 mm
$\frac{1}{1}$ + 3 mm

190

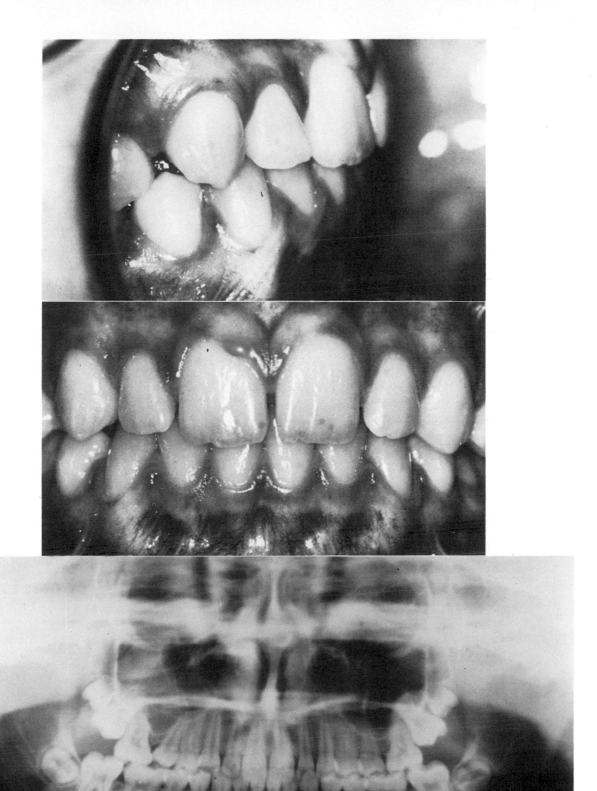

Fig. 181.   Patient N.G. after 3 years treatment. (a), (b) Photographs,
(c) orthopantomogram, (d) radiograph, (e) tracing.

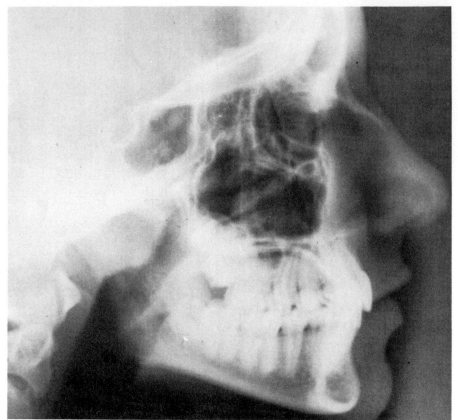

181d

181e N. G.
17. 7. 65
7. 2. 78

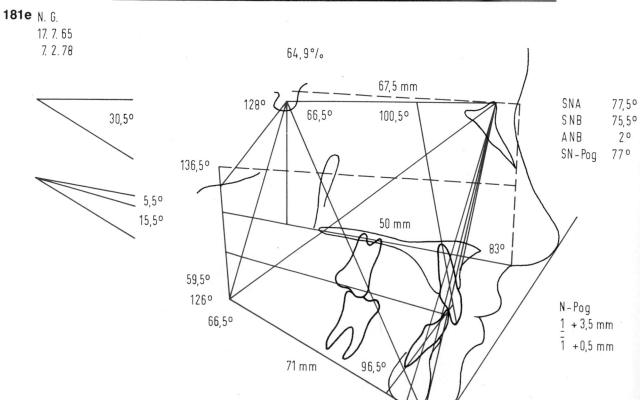

64,9 %

67,5 mm

128° 66,5° 100,5°

30,5°

136,5°

5,5°
15,5°

50 mm

83°

59,5°
126°

66,5°

71 mm   96,5°

SNA   77,5°
SNB   75,5°
ANB   2°
SN–Pog 77°

N–Pog
1 + 3,5 mm
1 + 0,5 mm

2.3 Distal Movement in the Maxilla

Headgear treatment to effect distal movement in the maxilla is indicated if the aim of treatment is to inhibit growth in the mid-face region. The method will often achieve a considerable reduction in the SNA angle. Cervical headgear therapy will effect distal movement and elevation of the teeth.

This form of treatment is, however, only possible when the direction of growth is not vertical; otherwise elevation of the molars would have an undesirable effect.

A 10-year-old girl (R.U.) presented with Class II$_1$ malocclusion, deep bite, and horizontal growth tendency (71.4%). There was marked convexity of the naso-maxillary complex (SNA angle 82°; Fig. 182a–e). The mandible was average in extent and well developed, its position posterior (SNB angle 75.5°). The small Go$_2$ angle (65°) and markedly horizontal direction of growth suggested that for the antero-posterior dental relationship the chances of correction were good, whilst those for opening the deep bite were poor.

This second and difficult problem was tackled first, the aim of treatment being also to inhibit growth in the maxillary region. Headgear therapy was initiated, and this was followed by activator treatment (Fig. 183a–e). After a treatment period of 3½ years including retention, the anomaly had been corrected, and the following changes were noted: The deep bite had been corrected despite the fact that the horizontal growth trend had increased. The SNA and SNB angles were within normal range (81° and 79°), with ANB 2°; the skeletal relationships had become normal. The maxillary and mandibular bases had increased by the normal annual growth rates. Growth in the vertical direction on the other hand had been above average, amounting to 9 mm in both posterior and anterior face height, i.e. 3 and 2 mm respectively above the average.

Upper incisor angulation and relationship to the NPog line had become normal. The lower incisors showed the right relationship to the NPog line, but still had a labial inclination of 104°. This labial inclination of the incisors had existed prior to treatment and was not corrected for the following reasons:

In view of adverse lip pressure, headgear therapy had been combined with a lower lip screen.

According to Schudy, the relationship of the lower incisors to the NPog line is a more important factor for stability than is their angulation.

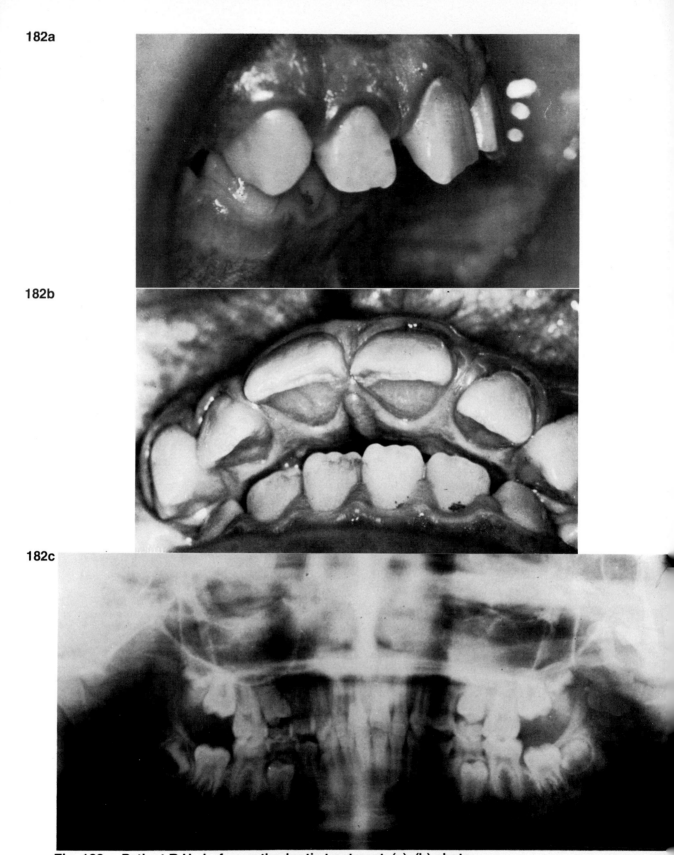

182a

182b

182c

Fig. 182. Patient R.U., before orthodontic treatment. (a), (b) photographs, (c) orthopantomogram, (d) radiograph, (e) tracing.

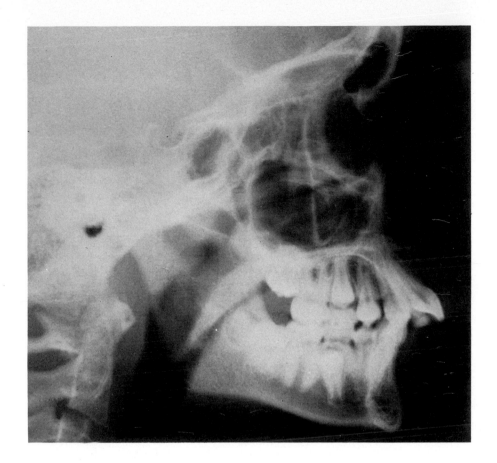

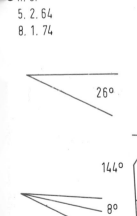

71,4 %

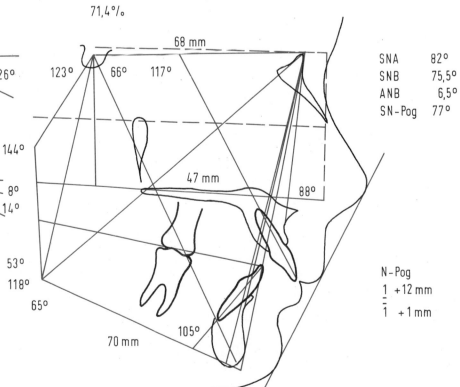

68 mm

26°   123°   66°   117°

144°

47 mm   88°

8°
14°

53°
118°

65°

105°

70 mm

SNA   82°
SNB   75,5°
ANB   6,5°
SN–Pog   77°

N–Pog
$\underline{1}$ +12 mm
$\overline{1}$ + 1 mm

183a

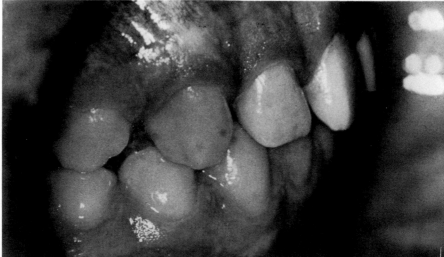

183b

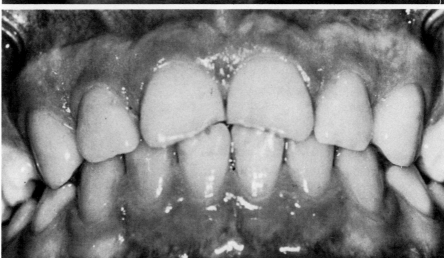

183c

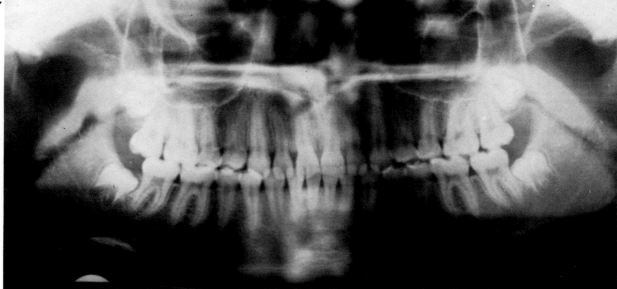

Fig. 183.   Patient R.U., after 3½ years orthodontic treatment. (a),
(b) Photographs, (c) orthopantomogram, (d) radiograph, (e) tracing.

196

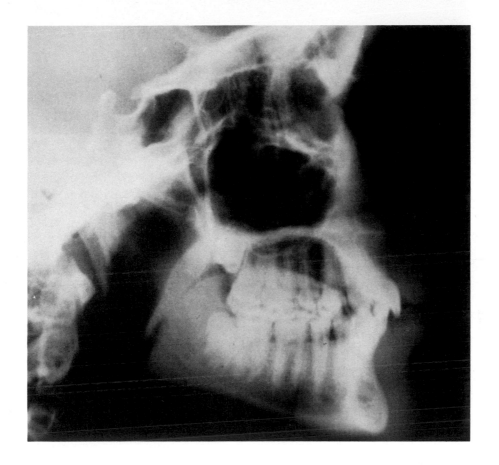

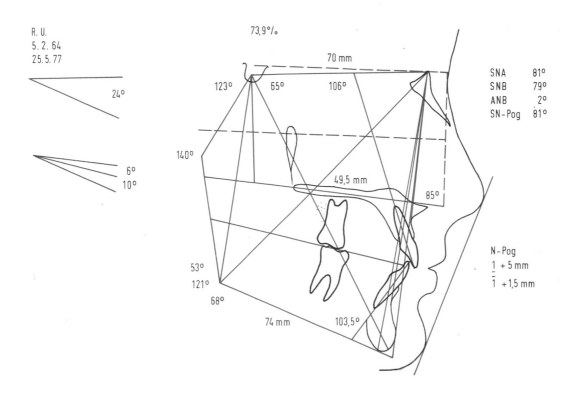

R. U.
5. 2. 64
25. 5. 77

24°

6°
10°

73,9 %

70 mm

123°   65°   106°

140°

49,5 mm

85°

53°
121°

68°

74 mm   103,5°

SNA   81°
SNB   79°
ANB   2°
SN-Pog   81°

N-Pog
1   + 5 mm
‾
1   + 1,5 mm

2.3.1   Headgear Therapy with Convexity of Nasomaxillary Complex

Convexity of the nasomaxillary complex is frequently the cause of a skeletal Class II relationship. The SNA angle is large in these cases, and ANS and Is1 are far anterior to the NPog line. Ante-inclination of the maxilla (large J angle) will increase protrusion, which A.M. Schwarz referred to as pseudo-protrusion. This ante-inclination arises through anterior swinging of the maxilla. The mid-face height (N-Sn) is short. In extreme cases Bimler speaks of microrhinal dysplasia. This form of Class II malocclusion can be corrected by cervical headgear therapy in mixed dentition, a pre-condition being that the direction of growth is not vertical.

A boy of 8 (G.Ch.) showed good development of the mandibular base, with prognathism. Class II malocclusion was due to forward displacement of the maxilla. Protrusion was enhanced by a 94° ante-inclination (pseudo-protrusion). After headgear therapy of almost 2 years duration, intermaxillary relations had become normal and the ANB angle was reduced from 10° to 2° (Fig. 184a, b; 185a, b).

A reduction in ANB by 8° is the maximum obtainable with headgear therapy. If treatment had started after the tenth year of life, a correction of this magnitude could not have been expected. Wieslander has shown in his follow-up studies that headgear therapy initiated during the eighth year gives very much better results than treatment given 18 months later (Fig. 186 and Table 20).

Changes in horizontal (⇄) or vertical (↑↓) direction	Early treatment	Late treatment	Difference
ANB	−3.24°	−1.84°	1.40°
6	3.13	1.43	1.70
Pogonion	0.12	0.37	0.49
ANS	↓5.40	↓3.69	1.71
Menton	↓9.73	↓7.33	2.40

Table 20.   Results achieved with headgear treatment given early (treatment started at age 8) and late (treatment started at age 10½) (Wieslander).

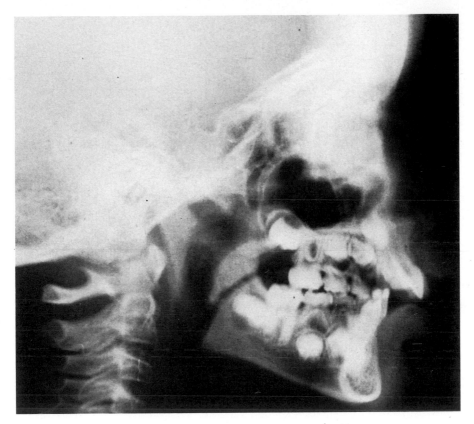

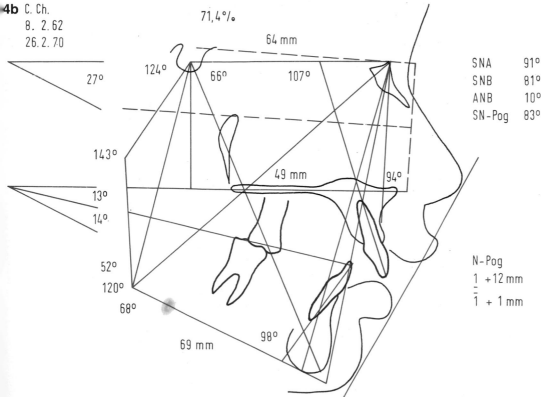

C. Ch.
8. 2.62
26.2.70

71,4 °/o

64 mm

124°   66°   107°

27°

143°

49 mm   94°

13°

14°

52°

120°

68°

69 mm   98°

SNA	91°
SNB	81°
ANB	10°
SN-Pog	83°

N-Pog

1 +12 mm

1 + 1 mm

Fig. 184. Eight-year-old boy, G.Ch., with prognathic profile and pseudoprotrusion, before orthodontic treatment. (a) Radiograph, (b) tracing.

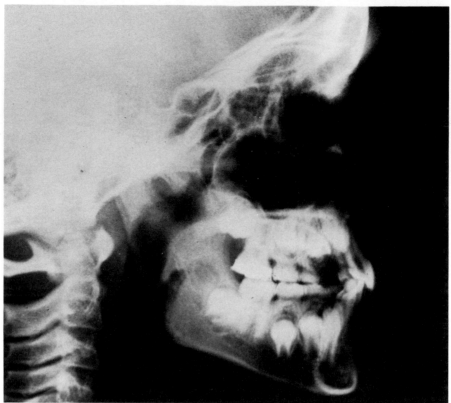

185a

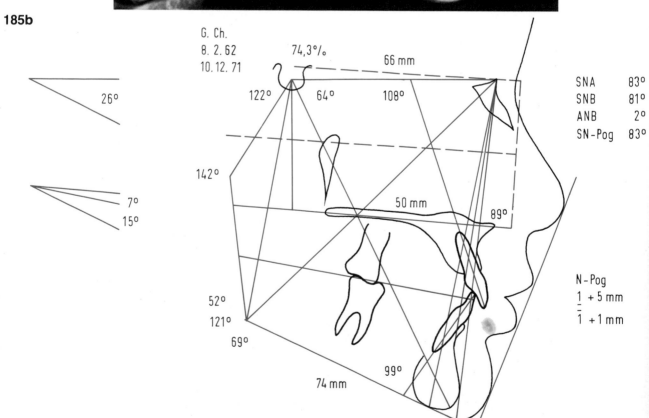

185b

Fig. 185. Patient G.Ch. after 2-year headgear therapy. (a) Radio-graph, (b) tracing.

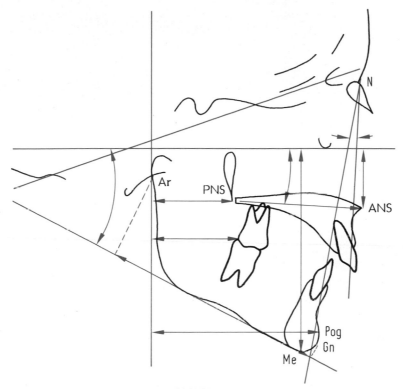

Fig. 186. Wieslander's cephalometric analysis to assess the results of headgear therapy.

2.4 Combined Therapy

A combination of headgear and subsequent activator therapy is frequently indicated with mid-face convexity and alveolar retroposition of the lower dental arch.

A 9-year-old boy (T.Ch.) presented with Class II₁ malocclusion including deep bite, adverse lip pressure and horizontal growth direction of 70% (Fig. 187a–g). The condition could be described as 'skeletal Class II malocclusion with the fault in the maxilla and dento-alveolar Class II malocclusion with the fault in the lower dental arch'. The SNA angle was 83°, SN-Pr 86°, the upper incisors protruded to 8 mm anterior to the NPog line. The mandibular position was normal, with an SNB angle of 79°.

The mandibular base was a little short (−3 mm), the ascending ramus was long (+3 mm). The lower incisors were very upright (86°) and 4 mm posterior to the NPog line. In the lower dental arch, there was practically no space for the canines. Analysis of the model indicated extraction therapy. Calculation of the discrepancy did, however, reveal that by moving the lower incisors forward it would still be possible to make space for the lower canines.

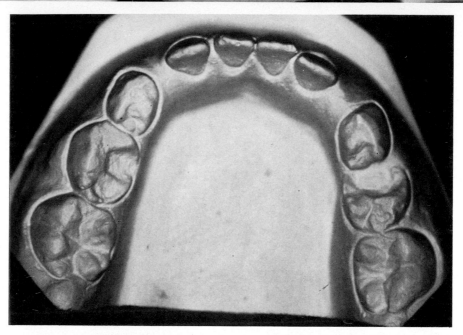

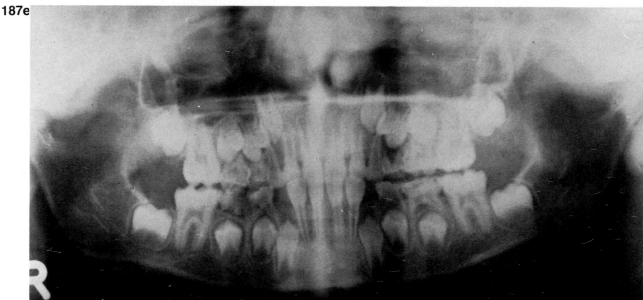

Fig. 187. Nine-year-old boy, T.Ch., with Class II₁ malocclusion, horizontal growth trend, and lip dysfunction, before orthodontic treatment. (a), (b), (c) Model, (d) lack of space for canines in the lower dental arch, (e) orthopantomogram, (f) radiograph, (g) tracing.

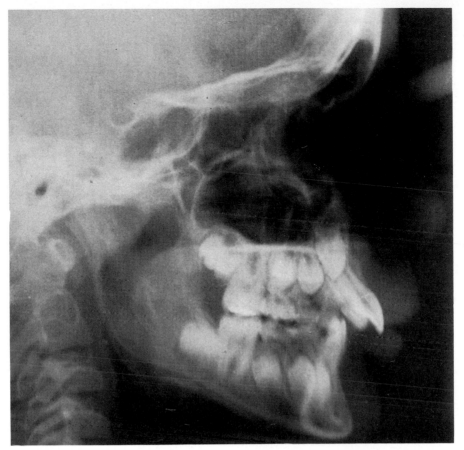

T. Ch.
16. 9. 64
27. 3. 73

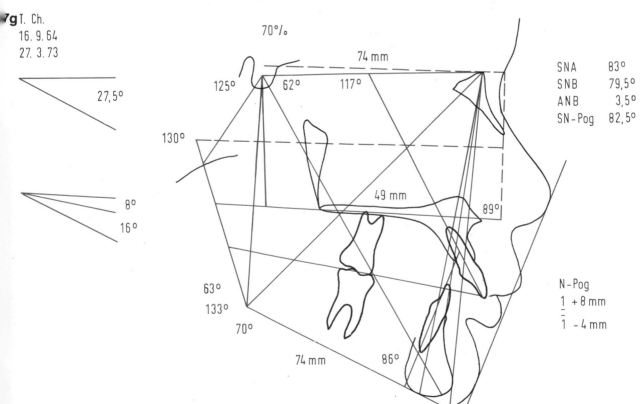

27,5°

8°
16°

63°
133°
70°

70‰

74 mm

125°   62°   117°

130°

49 mm   89°

74 mm   86°

SNA   83°
SNB   79,5°
ANB   3,5°
SN-Pog   82,5°

N-Pog
$\underline{1}$ + 8 mm
$\bar{\bar{1}}$ - 4 mm

203

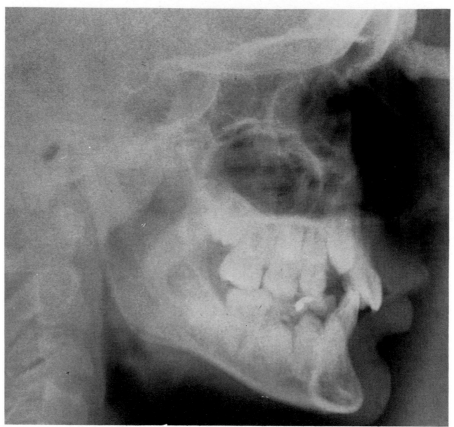

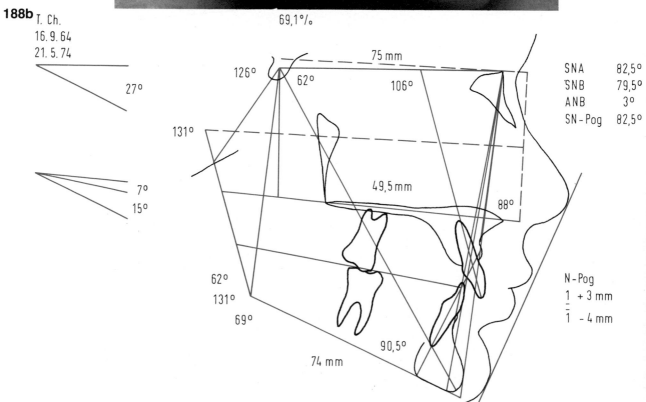

188a

69,1%

188b T. Ch.
16. 9. 64
21. 5. 74

27°

7°
15°

126°
62°
106°

131°

49,5mm

88°

62°
131°
69°

90,5°

74 mm

75 mm

SNA   82,5°
SNB   79,5°
ANB   3°
SN‑Pog 82,5°

N‑Pog
1̲ + 3 mm
1̄ − 4 mm

Fig. 188.   Intermediate result, after 1-year headgear therapy, patient T.Ch. (a) Radiograph, (b) tracing.

Treatment was initiated with headgear and a lower lip screen. After one year of treatment, the upper incisors had become established to a good relationship; the lower incisors had been uprighted, but were still 4 mm behind the NPog line (Fig. 188a, b).

Treatment then continued with an activator. The lower incisors were tipped forward, the canines showed good relationship. On conclusion of treatment the lower incisors were still 2 mm behind the NPog line, indicating that there was space in reserve (Fig. 189a–f).

a

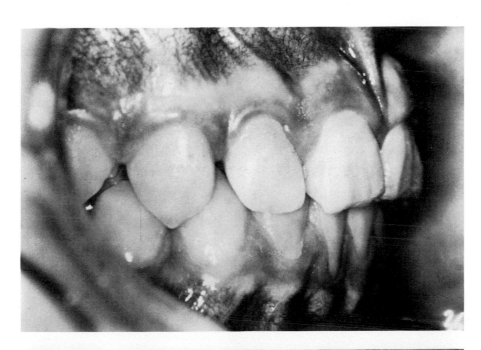

b

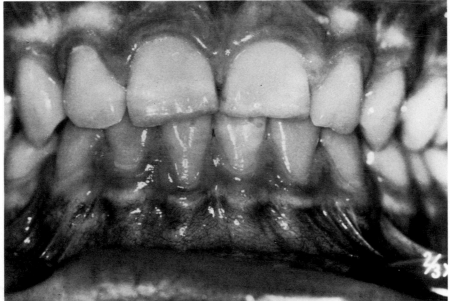

Fig. 189. Patient T.Ch., after activator therapy. (a), (b) Photographs, (c) canines well aligned in the lower dental arch, (d) orthopantomogram, (e) radiograph, (f) tracing.

189c

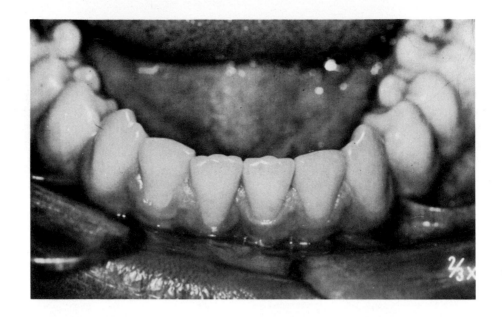

189d

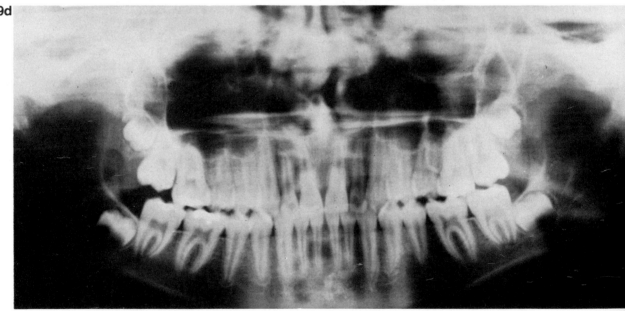

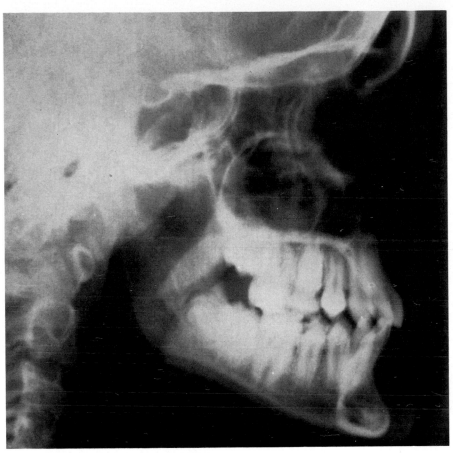

71,1%

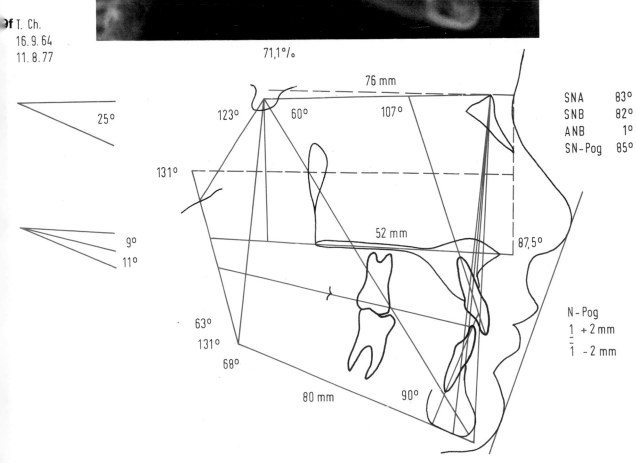

25°

123°   60°   107°

76 mm

131°

9°

11°

52 mm

87,5°

63°

131°

68°

80 mm   90°

SNA   83°
SNB   82°
ANB   1°
SN-Pog 85°

N-Pog
$\underline{1}$ + 2 mm
$\overline{1}$ − 2 mm

2.5 Discrepancy Calculation

The discrepancy gives the relationship of space available to space required. It may consist in too little space being available for the teeth in the lower dental arch, for instance. To determine whether the dental arch can be corrected without extraction or whether extraction will be necessary, the discrepancy has to be calculated. Model and radiographic relationships are used for the calculation, and distinction is made between:

(1) Dental discrepancy (DD), calculated on the model.

On the model, the clinical length of the dental arch is determined (from mesial 6 on the one side to mesial 6 on the other), taking into account crowding in front and the loss of space in the supporting zone for the cuspids and bicuspids. The difference between length of dental arch and place required for the dentition is the dental discrepancy (DD).

(2) Sagittal discrepancy (SD), calculated on the radiograph.

On the radiograph, the distance from the lower incisors (Is-1) to the NPog line is determined. This represents the sagittal discrepancy (SD). If the curve of Spee is exaggerated, 1–2 mm needs to be added to the sagittal discrepancy to make up for this.

(3) Total discrepancy (TD), a combination of the two.

The total discrepancy (TD) is the sum of the sagittal plus half the dental discrepancy as follows:

$$TD = SD + \tfrac{1}{2}DD$$

Treatment should be planned so that the lower incisors are no more than 4 mm anterior to the NPog line. If space is lacking in the model, it may be possible to gain space by protruding the lower incisors. Otherwise extraction therapy will be indicated. A total discrepancy of 7 mm for example would mean that a space of 7 mm was needed in each quadrant of the lower dental arch, which is practically the width of a premolar.

Interpretation of discrepancy in mixed dentition is subject, it will be remembered, to certain reservations, and further periods of active growth should be considered.

The principal results of model analysis and calculation of the discrepancy for patient T.Ch. are shown in Table 21.

		Maxilla		Mandible	
		SI$_o$: 36 mm		SI$_u$: 25 mm	
Supporting zone	Ideal	23.7 mm		23.4 mm	
	Found	r. 26.5	l. 25.5	r. 22.0	l. 22.0
	Diff.	+2.8	+1.8	−1.4	−1.4
Length of dental arch	Ideal	21 mm		19 mm	
	Found	25 mm		14 mm	
	Diff.	+4 mm		−5 mm	

Space available: 36 mm

Space required: 39 mm DD $= \dfrac{-3-1}{2} = -2$

For the curve of Spee 1 mm is required.

Distance of lower incisors from NPog: −4 mm SD = +6 mm

Discrepancy: −2(DD)+6(SD) = +4 mm(TD)

Table 21. Principal data in model analysis of patient T.Ch.

3 Late Treatment

With horizontal growth trends, the possibility of changing the antero-posterior skeletal relationship also depends on a fourth dimension, the time factor. Once active growth has ceased, correction of malocclusions is possible only with regard to translocated closures. Treatment becomes limited to distal movement of the upper teeth. Again diagnosis and treatment planning are largely dependent on analysis of the radiograph.

In the case of B.A., a girl aged 15, the Class II malocclusion with deep bite and horizontal growth direction could be corrected only in the dento-alveolar region (Fig. 190a–f), skeletal correction being no longer possible at that age. The facial skeleton was prognathic, with an SNA angle of 85°, and SNB angle of 82°. The mandible was well developed, and 7 mm above average in length. She presented with Class II malocclusion, the fault being in the maxilla. In view also of her age, distal movement of the upper teeth was the only feasible treatment. The upper incisors were tipped labially, and 8 mm anterior to the NPog line. The lower incisors showed correct angulation and normal position relative to the line. Distal movement of the upper teeth with intermaxillary anchorage was indicated. The aim in a case of this type must be to keep the mandibular incisors in their existing position, merely levelling the compensatory curve, and to effect distal movement of the upper teeth. This would be the only means of correcting the deep bite as well as the distocclusion. The horizontal growth trend contra-indicated extraction of the premolars, as that would make correction of the deep bite impossible. To establish the correct relationship of upper and lower incisors, it was necessary to effect distal movement of the whole upper dental arch. If the germs of the wisdom teeth are present, extraction of the upper 12th-year molars is indicated in these cases.

190a   190b   190c

190d

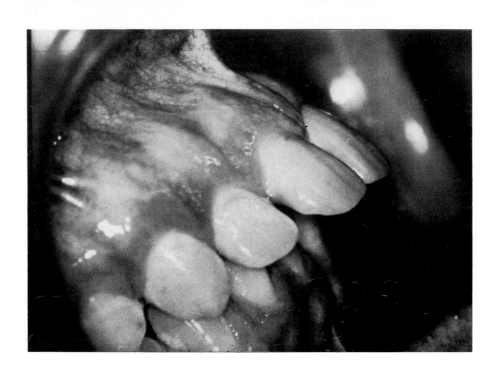

Fig. 190.   Girl aged 15, B.A., before orthodontic treatment. (a), (b), (c) Model, (d) photograph showing small apical base in the maxilla, (e) radiograph, (f) tracing.

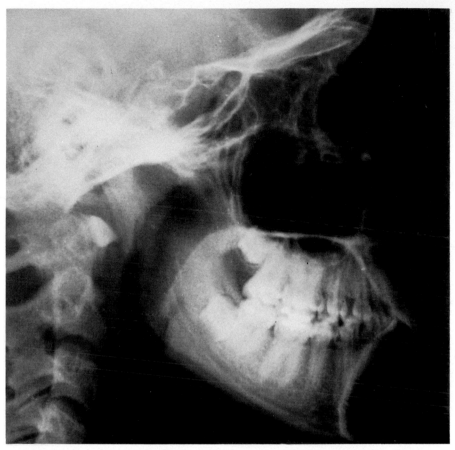

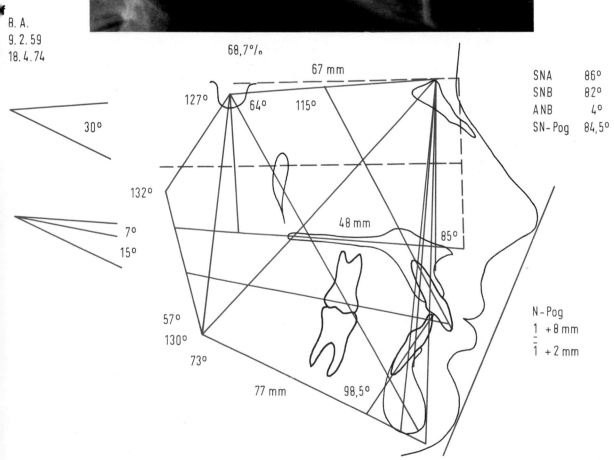

B. A.
9. 2. 59
18. 4. 74

68,7%

67 mm

127°   64°   115°

30°

132°

7°
15°

48 mm

85°

57°
130°

73°

77 mm   98,5°

SNA   86°
SNB   82°
ANB   4°
SN-Pog 84,5°

N-Pog
1   +8 mm
1   +2 mm

After a 3-year period of treatment and retention, the Class II malocclusion had been corrected by dento-alveolar changes. The skeletal relationships had remained unchanged. The lower incisors were maintained in position, the upper dental arch had been moved distally, and the deep bite fully corrected. No appreciable growth changes were noted (Fig. 191a–d).

Apart from establishing the indication, cephalometric radiography is also required in cases where active growth has ceased, to plan the anchorage requirement, decide on the form incisor movement should take, and to monitor the results.

191a

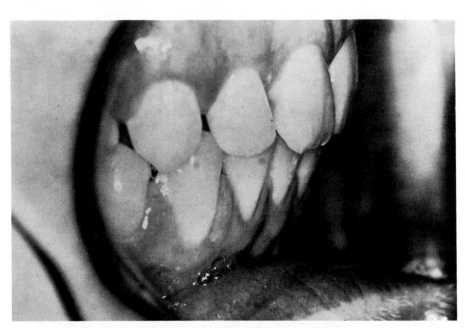

191b

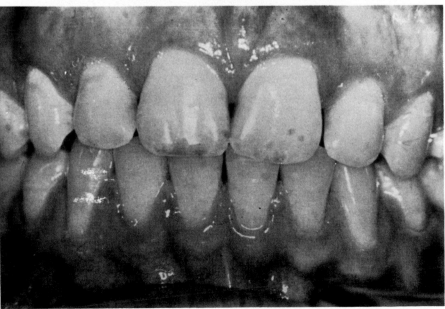

Fig. 191. Patient B.A., after orthodontic treatment. (a), (b) Photographs, (c) radiograph, (d) tracing.

c

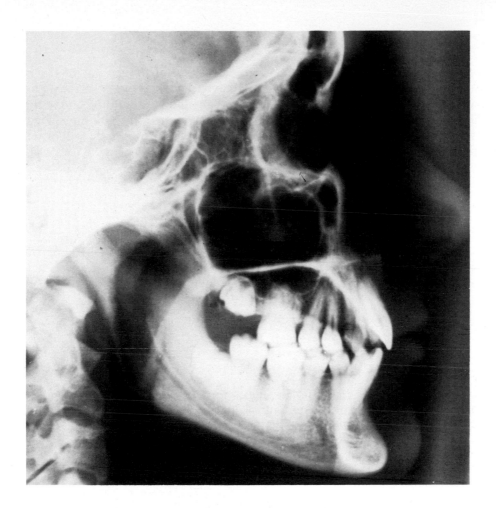

d

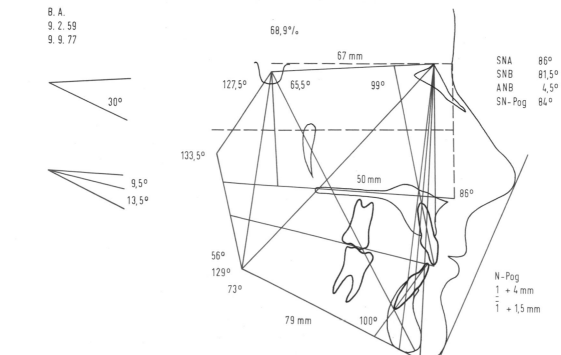

B. A.
9. 2. 59
9. 9. 77

68,9 %

67 mm

127,5°   65,5°   99°

SNA   86°
SNB   81,5°
ANB   4,5°
SN-Pog   84°

30°

133,5°

50 mm

86°

9,5°
13,5°

56°
129°
73°

79 mm   100°

N-Pog
$\underline{1}$ + 4 mm
$\overline{1}$ + 1,5 mm

213

3.1 Planning the Anchorage

When distocclusion is corrected at a late stage, distal movement of the upper dentition requires rather heavy forces. We have to consider very seriously how to apply these forces in keeping with our anchoring values. Depending on the form of anchorage used, distinction is made between three degrees of anchorage (Fig. 192). The form of anchorage used depends largely on whether treatment will or will not include extraction.

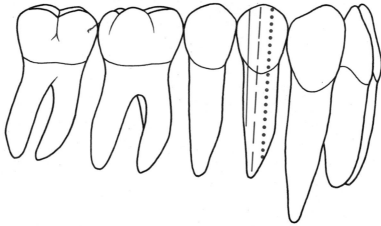

Fig. 192. Available space for mandibular anchorage. The dotted line indicates the limit for mesial movement of anchor teeth with minimal anchorage; the broken line shows the anterior limit of mesial movement for the anchor teeth with moderate anchorage; the solid line shows the limit with maximum anchorage.

(1) *Minimal anchorage:* The force applied may be reciprocal.

(a) Spaces left after extraction are to ¾ closed from distal, and only to ¼ from mesial.

(b) The lower incisors are very upright and behind the NPog line, the lower dental arch is well aligned.

(2) *Moderate anchorage:* The force applied can no longer be reciprocal, the load on the anchor teeth must be distributed, or their resistance needs to be reinforced.

(a) Spaces gained by extraction can be closed to between ½ and ¼ from distal, and between ½ and ¾ from mesial.

(b) Calculation of the total discrepancy shows that, after treatment, the lower incisors will be a maximum of 2–4 mm anterior to the NPog line.

Reciprocal intramaxillary anchorage is contra-indicated in this group. Inter-maxillary anchorage will usually be suitable (though contra-indicated with vertical growth trends).

(3) *Maximum anchorage:* No space must be lost from the distal side in the anchorage area, and anchorage must therefore be stationary.

(a) The spaces provided by extraction must be closed from mesial.

(b) Calculation of the discrepancy shows that the lower incisors are 4 mm anterior to the NPog line (with antero-position greater than that, extraction is usually indicated). Anchorage needs to be reinforced by extra-oral traction (headgear in maxilla or mandible).

In the case of our patient B.A., the dental discrepancy was 1.5 mm, sagittal discrepancy 0 mm, and total discrepancy, after aligning the curve of Spee, 2 mm. A total discrepancy of 2 mm allows very little room for anchor movement, and maximum anchorage is required. In this case, it was reinforced with headgear in the mandible (Fig. 193).

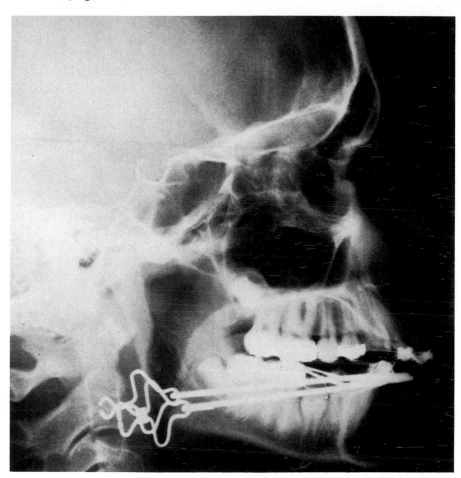

Fig. 193.   Headgear in the mandible, with maximum anchorage.

4   Correction of Class II₁ Malocclusions with Vertical Growth Direction

Certain aspects require special consideration when treating a Class II₁ malocclusion with vertical growth trend. Correction of deep bite usually presents no problems in this group, but with antero-posterior occlusal relationships there are certain reservations. Distal movement and extrusion of the buccal teeth will enhance mandibular retrognathism. Extraction of the first premolars on the other hand is indicated, as mesial movement of the buccal teeth will weaken the vertical growth trend. It is sometimes also possible to extract the premolars in the upper arch only, with no risk of deep bite developing.

Taking into account the skeletal features of these cases, we have developed a special activator for correction of Class II malocclusion with vertical growth trends, the 'V' (vertical) activator (Fig. 194). This utilises the forces of the musculature more in the vertical and less in the horizontal direction. We achieve this by using a high working bite for the activator, without bringing the mandible massively forward (Fig. 195a, b). This position increases myostatic reflex activity and utilises the visco-elastic properties of the soft tissues for the application of force. The muscle force thus produced is more intensive and of greater duration than with activators designed to use swallowing as the chief source of power. The 'V' activator is rigid in construction in order to evoke isometric muscle contractions which again are longer in duration than those developed with an elastic activator.

194

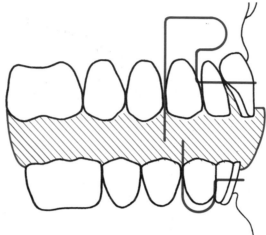

Fig. 194.   Diagram showing vertical activator with high working bite.

195a

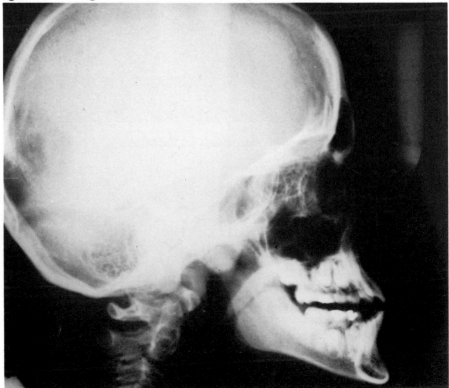

Fig. 195.   Construction bite (a) with horizontal growth type, (b) with vertical growth type.

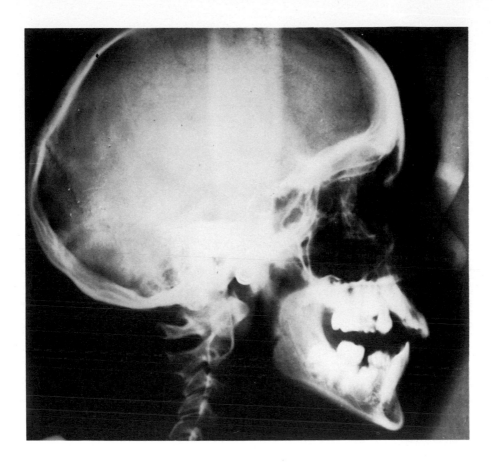

Cephalometric radiography is of vital importance, not only in establishing the indication for this construction of the activator, but also when the working bite is taken, as not only the direction of growth and functional relationships, but also the inclination of the mandible and mandibular plane and the position and axial inclination of the incisors needs to be taken into account.

A bite chamfer anteriorly ground into the acrylic to hold or support the upper incisors is frequently added to a 'V' activator. This construction enhances the growth inhibiting effect in the maxillary area (Fig. 196).

Patients with a vertical type of facial skeleton do not tolerate massive forward movement of the mandible by the appliance. It would certainly be wrong to treat with growth and not take the growth pattern into account. A vertically raised activator will bring the mandible slightly forward and downward, with simultaneous adaption of the maxilla to the lower dental arch.

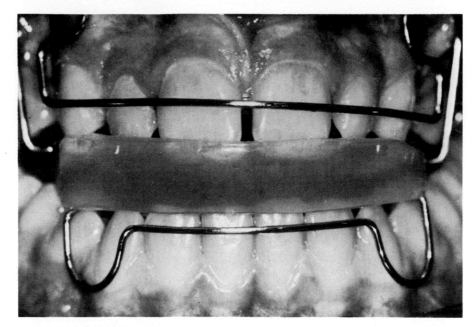

Fig. 196. Frontal support with vertical activator.

A 9-year-old boy, G.F., presented with Class II₁ malocclusion, tongue and lip dysfunction, and lip incompetence. The direction of growth was vertical, at 55%, and the sum of angles 406° (Fig. 197a–e). The gonial angle was not large, with 125°, but the lower Go₂ angle was greatly enlarged, at 78°. The ascending ramus was short (−10 mm), the maxillary and mandibular bases showed normal development. The facial skeleton was retrognathic, SNA being 77°, and SNB 71°. Incisor angulation was normal, with the upper incisors 12 mm anterior to the facial plane.

Treatment therefore had to achieve the following:

(1) Inhibit the sagittal growth trend in the maxilla, rotate it downwards and move both 6 year molars in the distal direction.

(2) Bring the mandible slightly forward and down, with slight forward rotation. The active growth phases that lay ahead were to be utilised for this purpose.

The 'V' activator permits distalisation of the two 6 year molars with fixation pins, and the upper front to be supported to enable anterior-inferior rotation of the maxilla towards the mandible. With a carefully planned working bite and selective grinding of the activator, it is possible to encourage anterior and superior rotation of the mandible.

197a 197b 197c

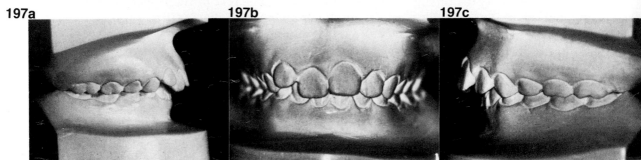

Fig. 197. Patient G.F., vertical face type, before orthodontic treatment. (a), (b), (c) Models, (d) radiograph, (e) tracing.

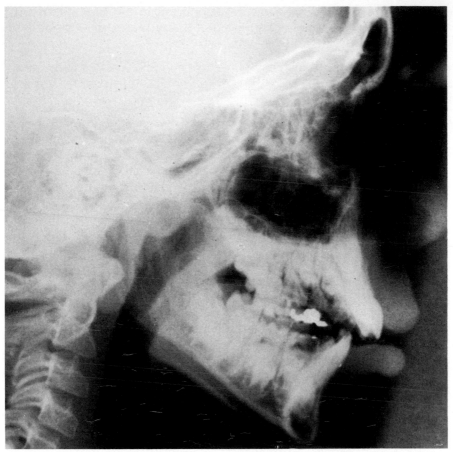

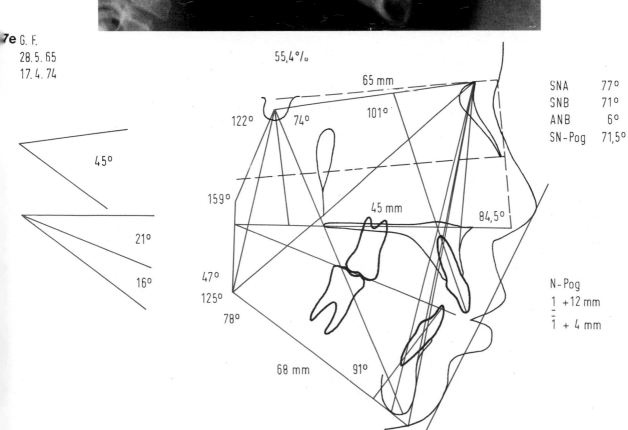

7e G. F.
28. 5. 65
17. 4. 74

55,4 %

65 mm

122°   74°   101°

45°

159°

45 mm

84,5°

21°

16°

47°
125°

78°

68 mm   91°

SNA   77°
SNB   71°
ANB   6°
SN-Pog   71,5°

N-Pog
$\underline{1}$ +12 mm
$\overline{1}$ + 4 mm

With treatment continued for a three year period in the case of patient G.F., active growth phases and the eruption potential of the teeth were utilised. The following changes were noted (Fig. 198a–d).

In the *maxilla*, inclination was reduced by 3.5°, and SNA by 1°; the maxillary base gained 1.5 mm through growth. Rotation was achieved as planned, with growth inhibited.

The *mandible* rotated upwards and forward, with a change in direction of growth from 55% to 58%. The gonial angle increased, but Go_2 was reduced, again through rotation of the mandible. The mandibular base had grown by 7 mm, the SNB angle increased by 2°, whilst the ANB angle had decreased from 6° to 3°. Mutual rotation of the maxillary and mandibular bases served to restore normal occlusion.

198a

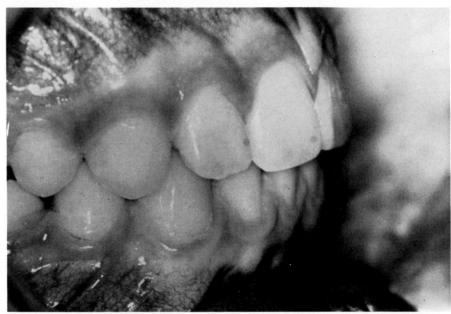

198b

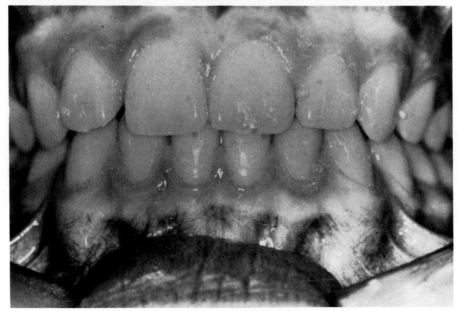

Fig. 198. **Patient G.F. after three years of treatment with vertical activator. (a), (b) Photographs, (c) radiograph, (d) tracing.**

c

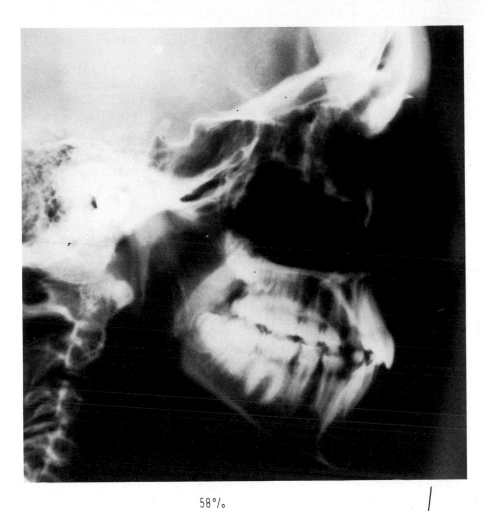

d G. F.
28.5.65
16.8.77

58%

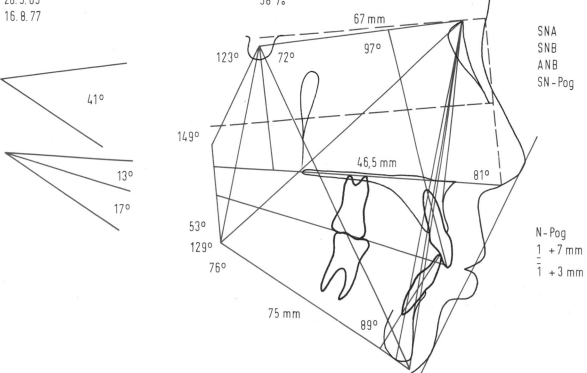

41°

13°

17°

123°   72°   97°

67 mm

149°

46,5 mm

81°

53°
129°
76°

75 mm   89°

SNA   76°
SNB   73°
ANB   3°
SN–Pog   74°

N–Pog
$\frac{1}{}$ + 7 mm
$\frac{\overline{1}}{}$ + 3 mm

The Ranking Order of Cephalometric Radiography in Orthodontic Diagnosis

Cephalometric radiography was introduced into orthodontics by Broadbent and Brodie and by Hofrath in 1930. For many years, however, treatment continued to be given without benefit of cephalometrics, and it was not until the 60s that it gradually gained acceptance in daily practice. Sceptics would be right to ask, therefore, if it is not merely a passing fashion.

The real need for cephalometrics in orthodontic diagnosis has arisen with the development of orthodontic therapy. In the old days, 'universal' appliances were generally used. There were activator 'schools' and plate 'schools', and diagnostic methods were not very demanding.

Today, not only are different methods used, but various methods are even used in combination during different stages of treatment for the same patient. This calls for accurate differential diagnosis and continuous diagnostic monitoring. High quality treatment means that sophisticated methods of diagnosis will also have to be used.

In an age of ergonomics, the time factor tends to be a major problem. Making a tracing and the required measurements is time-consuming. Can this task be delegated? Accurate localisation of reference points is a pre-condition for a reliable analysis, and this demands knowledge of anatomy and X-ray anatomy. This task, i.e. the localisation of reference points, should not be delegated. Joining up the points and measuring out distances and angles, on the other hand, can be left to assistants given requisite training. The interpretation of the results is one of the most important stages in the analysis, and can only be done by the orthodontist himself as major decisions are based on this interpretation.

How far can modern technology assist us? Apparatus for the semi-automatic determination of angles and distances is available. These machines are known as cephalometric tracers or digitisers. Their interpretation, and the choice of treatment are, however, the task of the orthodontist.

The system known as computer diagnosis, with complete treatment plans and all decisions provided by automatic machines, is too rigid a system, and it is only programmed for specific methods of treatment. In medicine, too, it has been the experience that the final decision and logical analysis remains the function of the physician.

A common problem in producing the radiograph is the linear distance from tube target to subject. A distance of four metres will produce practically no enlargement. In daily practice this is, however, not usually feasible. Taking radiographs from a great distance presents problems of both space and finance. Space is required to install the unit, and a high-power four-valve apparatus has to be acquired. Smaller units are therefore generally used, with a distance of 1½ metres between film and object. The angular values will be practically the same as with 4 metre radiographs. Linear dimensions need correction by about 6% before they are interpreted. The 1½ metre units certainly make it easier to introduce cephalometrics into daily practice.

Cephalometric radiography enables us to analyse the facial skeleton for treatment planning and serves as a reliable guide as treatment progresses.

The more demanding forms of treatment cannot today be envisaged without cephalometric radiography, but even with 'simple' anomalies, the method offers security against misjudgement.

Appendix
Case Sheet. Cephalometric Analysis of patient T.Ch. (continuous diagnosis)

Name: T.Ch.	*Freiburg Analysis*				
d.o.b. 16.09.64		I	II	III	IV
	Norm	27.3.73	21.5.74	21.1.76	11.8.77
NS–Ar (saddle angle)	123°+5°	125	126	125	123
S–ArGo (articular angle)	143°∓6°	130	131	132	131
Ar–GoMe (gonial angle)	130°∓7°	133	131	130	131
Sum: Horiz. growth / Vert. growth	396°	388	388	387	385
Go₁ (upper) Ar–Go–N	52–55°	63	62	61	63
Go₂ (lower) NGo²–Me	70–75°	70	69	69	68
SNA	81°	83	82.5	82	83
SNB	79°	79.5	79.5	81	82
ANB	2°	3.5	3	1	1
SN–prosthion	84°	86	84	84	85.5
SN–infradentale	81°	80	79.5	81.5	83.5
SN–Pog	80°	82.5	82.5	84	85
Pal–MeGo (basal ∢)	25°	24	22	22	20
Pal–Occ	11°	8	7	6	9
MeGo–Occ	14°	16	15	16	11
SN–MeGo	32°	27.5	27	27	25
SeN–Pal (∢ of incl.)	85°	89	88	87	87.5
NS–Gn (Y axis)	66°	62	62	61	60
S–Go: NMe x 100	62–65%	70%	69.1%	69.2%	71.1%
		73,5:105	74:107	76:109	79:111

Name: T.Ch.	*Freiburg Analysis*				
d.o.b. 16.09.64		I	ii	iii	iv
	Norm	27.3.73	21.5.74	21.1.76	11.8.77
1 SN	102°±2°	117	106	106	107
1 Pal (Schwarz)	70°±5°	59.5	69.5	69	68
1 MeGo (posterior)	90°±3°	86	90.5	94	90
NPog to 1	2–4mm	+8	+3	+1.5	+2
NPog to 1	−2−+2mm	−4	−4	−2	−2
Inter-incisal angle	135°	130	136	134	136.5
S–Ar	35mm	34.5	36	38	39
NSe (+3mm = mandible)	74–49–53	75–50–53.5	75–50–53.5	76–50.5–60	
Mand./maxilla/asc.r length/ramus width	74–49–56	74–49.5–56	78–51.5–57	80–52–45	
Symphysis	thick thin normal	thick	thick	thick	thick
S′–F.Ptp	14–15mm	17	17	14.5	16.5
SS′	42–57mm	41	42	42.5	45
Distance to aesthetic line labrale sup.	−1 to −4mm	+1	0	−2.5	−2
labrale inf.	0 to +2mm	−1	−1	−3	−3

Other details:

Bibliography

1. *Andrews, L. F.:* The six keys to normal occlusion. Am. J. Orthod. 62: 296–309, 1972
2. *Björk, A.; Skieller, V.:* Facial development and tooth eruption. Am. J. Orthod. 62: 339–383, 1972
3. *Broadbent, B. H.; Golden, W. H.:* Bolton standards of dentofacial development growth. Mosby, St. Louis 1975
4. *Greulich, W. W.; Pyle, S. J.:* Radiographic atlas of skeletal development of the hand and wrist. Stanford University Press, Stanford 1970
5. *Holdaway, R. A.:* The "V.T.O.". The University of Texas Press, Houston 1976
6. *Jarabak, J. R.; Fizzel, J. A.:* Light-wire edgewise Appliance. Mosby, St. Louis 1972
7. *Krogman, W. M.; Sassouni, V.:* Syllabus in Roentgenographic Cephalometry. Center of Research in Child growth. Philadelphia 1957
8. *Rakosi, Th.:* Die Fernröntgenanalyse. Die Funktionsanalyse. Leitfaden für Fortbildungskurse, Freiburg 1973
9. *Ricketts, R. M.:* The value of cephalometrics and computerized technology. Angle Orthod. 42: 179–199, 1972
10. *Riolo, M. L.; Moyers, R. W.; McNamara, J. A.; Hunter, W. S.:* An atlas of craniofacial growth. Center of human growth and development. Ann Arbor 1974
11. *Schwarz, A. M.:* Die Röntgenostatik. Urban & Schwarzenberg, Wien 1958

Index